GEORGE M. ARNOLD, M.D.

FEEL
YOUR BEST
LIVE
YOUR BEST

A NATURAL RETURN *to*
HORMONE BALANCE

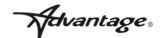

Published by Advantage, Charleston, South Carolina.
Member of Advantage Media Group.

ADVANTAGE is a registered trademark, and the Advantage colophon is a trademark of Advantage Media Group, Inc.

Printed in the United States of America.

10 9 8 7 6 5 4 3 2 1

ISBN: 978-1-59932-816-4
LCCN: 2017950355

Cover design by George Stevens.
Layout design by Megan Elger.

This publication is designed to provide accurate and authoritative information in regard to the subject matter covered. It is sold with the understanding that the publisher is not engaged in rendering legal, accounting, or other professional services. If legal advice or other expert assistance is required, the services of a competent professional person should be sought.

Advantage Media Group is proud to be a part of the Tree Neutral® program. Tree Neutral offsets the number of trees consumed in the production and printing of this book by taking proactive steps such as planting trees in direct proportion to the number of trees used to print books. To learn more about Tree Neutral, please visit **www.treeneutral.com.**

Advantage Media Group is a publisher of business, self-improvement, and professional development books. We help entrepreneurs, business leaders, and professionals share their Stories, Passion, and Knowledge to help others Learn & Grow. Do you have a manuscript or book idea that you would like us to consider for publishing? Please visit **advantagefamily.com** or call **1.866.775.1696.**

This book is dedicated to my best friend and wife, Bimpe,
who "feels her best and lives her best" every day and encourages
not only me but also everyone to do the same.

GEORGE ARNOLD, M.D.

George Arnold, MD, completed his medical training at the University of Toronto in 1986. Following a year as a family and emergency physician, he returned to the University of Toronto to complete his specialty training in obstetrics and gynecology. He has been in practice as an obstetrician/gynecologist since 1992.

A highly regarded and sought-after physician with patients from around the world, Dr. Arnold has extensive skill and experience when it comes to women's hormone issues. A part of his practice is now devoted to treating hormone imbalances.

Dr. Arnold is known as a kind, caring physician who listens to a patient's concerns and then works with the patient to identify the cause of symptoms. In addition to treating perimenopausal and menopausal symptoms, Dr. Arnold has experience with thyroid disorders and adrenal fatigue.

As more women—and men—take control of their own health and seek out clinics and practitioners to work with, it is important to select someone with a proven record of success.

Table of Contents

Acknowledgments

I would like to thank all my patients who have encouraged me to write this book. It is they who have challenged me to find natural solutions for their problems, and once those were fixed, to expand my practice to treat their partners as well. My patients continue to be a source of tremendous encouragement to me.

I would also like to thank the Advantage Media team for their tremendous support and dedication. Their high standards have resulted in an outstanding educational resource that I trust will be a blessing and help to everyone who reads it.

WELCOME TO "THE BEST-ME CLUB"

Too often, women suffer in silence. They feel they're the only one experiencing the symptoms of perimenopause or menopause.

But you're not alone. You're part of a large community of women who are experiencing similar symptoms and are at a similar place in their lives.

There's help available. In my practice, rather than just treating symptoms, our emphasis is on identifying the cause of your symptoms, and then we custom tailor solutions to suit your specific hormone-replacement needs in order to restore balance to your life. Just as you are unique, your treatment should be unique to you.

Since you're reading this book, you are already on track to improve your health. You're one of the thousands of women—and now men, too—who are experiencing problems with their health but know there's a solution out there. That solution is natural hormone-replacement therapy, also known as *bioidentical hormones*.

Bioidentical hormones are extracted from natural sources, such as plants like soybeans and yams. Their molecular structure is identical to that of the hormones produced within our own bodies.

ABOUT ME

I've been in practice since 1992. In the first few years, I saw a lot of women who were having side effects from one of the common hormone treatments at that time, Premarin. That had me looking for alternatives that would help with women's symptoms and not have the same side effects.

My journey eventually led me to use bioidentical hormones, something I like to call *nature's replacement therapy*. I've been amazed at the improvements I've seen in patients using these natural hormones. I'm a firm believer that all hormones in the body should work together, and I've devoted a part of my practice to treating hormone imbalances.

Today, there is greater awareness of bioidentical hormones through promotion by people in the entertainment industry. That has led many patients to consider them more, to research solutions that might be best for them, and to see, as a result, that bioidentical hormones are safe and that there are many benefits to using them.

As a result, I've had more patients come to me showing an interest in using them—both women and men.

But there are still a lot of people who don't realize that bioidentical hormones are the answer to the problems that they're experiencing.

WHO IS THIS BOOK FOR?

The majority of patients I treat are women in the menopausal age group with symptoms of hot flashes, night sweats, difficulty sleeping, and mood disruption—especially feeling down. They'll see the silliest little thing on TV and just dissolve in tears. They realize that the way they're reacting isn't normal, but they don't have any control over their emotions. They'll complain of decreased interest in sex. They'll have difficulty concentrating. They are much more irritable, and they aren't able to multitask. They'll find that they're starting to put on weight, especially around the midsection, and that their energy is down.

I wrote this book primarily for women forty-five to sixty years old who are beyond their childbearing years. However, since natural hormones are also used in fertility treatment, I'm also including information for women who are struggling with pregnancy issues. I also treat men, because women I've helped significantly with hormones often want their partners to experience the same improvements they've had. Therefore, each chapter will also contain a bit of information for men as well.

Most people I see as patients are experiencing various symptoms and want to have them treated in a natural way—meaning if hormone replacement is the treatment solution, then they want natural or bioidentical medications. Some patients recognize that their symptoms are due to menopause. They've either read about and recognize their symptoms, or they have a friend who's been through the same thing. In fact, many new patients are referred by my current patients. They see the difference natural hormones have made in the life of a friend, and they want to experience the same thing for themselves.

I'm also going to share patient stories throughout this book in hopes that you may see someone's situation as similar to your own and possibly realize that bioidentical hormones are a viable treatment option for you as well. In these stories, I've changed the names of patients to protect their identities.

If you see yourself in one of these stories, or if you've just felt a few changes in your body and know that things aren't quite right—and your current doctor is telling you that "it's old age, get used to it"—then read on. I think you'll be pleasantly surprised to find that you don't have to just "live with it" when changes occur during the latter half of your life that interfere with your ability to "feel your best and live your best."

SYMPTOM CHART

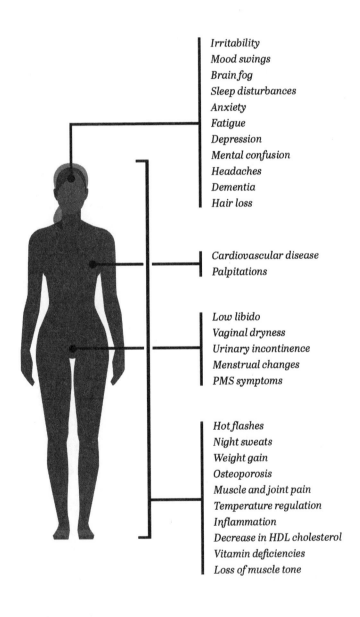

Irritability
Mood swings
Brain fog
Sleep disturbances
Anxiety
Fatigue
Depression
Mental confusion
Headaches
Dementia
Hair loss

Cardiovascular disease
Palpitations

Low libido
Vaginal dryness
Urinary incontinence
Menstrual changes
PMS symptoms

Hot flashes
Night sweats
Weight gain
Osteoporosis
Muscle and joint pain
Temperature regulation
Inflammation
Decrease in HDL cholesterol
Vitamin deficiencies
Loss of muscle tone

At age forty-nine, Jane started to experience hot flashes and night sweats. She would fall asleep and wake at three in the morning staring at the ceiling, only to fall back to sleep at six a.m. just in time to be woken by her alarm. A well-known CEO, she found herself turning beet red and becoming drenched in sweat in the middle of business meetings. She found herself increasingly short-tempered and forgetting things that were routine. Her razor-sharp memory was becoming quite dull, and her work performance was slipping.

At age forty-five, Robert began experiencing decreased energy, poor sleep, and increased anxiety. He felt "wired" all the time. His symptoms became so incapacitating that he had to step away from his real estate business.

At age forty-eight, Alison was noticing a big increase in fatigue. Her periods were becoming much heavier and lasting longer. Her coworkers found her irritable and less productive. Her own sense of well-being had more or less disappeared.

At age sixteen, Nicole's anxiety had become so severe that she had not been able to attend school for two years, and she had trouble even leaving the house. Her symptoms started at the same time her period did and had gradually worsened.

At age sixteen, Angela was feeling a constant loss of energy and experiencing worsening anxiety and depression.

At age fourteen, Amanda was tired all the time, she had difficulty sleeping, and she was always getting sick. She was missing a lot of school as a result.

At age forty-eight, Erin had begun noticing changes in her body. In addition to irregular menstrual cycles, she was gaining weight in spite of her workouts. Over time, she noticed her nails becoming more brittle, and her hairbrush seemed to come away with more strands every time she used it. She even began to lose hair in her eyebrows, and over time, she found she had to shave her legs less often. More and more she felt cold, and her bones and joints ached—but she had written off her symptoms to a chronic cold and arthritis.

At age forty-seven, Jane found herself increasingly depressed and feeling anxious about everyday things that were likely not to be a problem—bills coming due, meeting deadlines, the car breaking down. She was having trouble with her sex drive—to the frustration of her and her husband—and she was beginning to lose sleep. Her menstrual cycle had begun to be sporadic, causing her further frustration.

At age thirty-four, Louise became pregnant with her second child. She had experienced mild postpartum depression following her first delivery three years prior but had taken no medication for the condition at that time. However, during her week-thirty visit to my office, she began complaining of worsening depression.

In her midfifties, Sam had already been "feeling her age." She'd already been dealing with what she decided were probably symptoms of menopause—hot flashes, night sweats, and increasing moodiness. Then she began feeling more fatigued and was having a lot of trouble maintaining her concentration at work, changes she chalked up to what had become a sporadic sleep pattern at best. When her hair started thinning at an alarming rate, she went to see her family physician, who offered no solution and just wanted to prescribe a sedative to help her sleep at night. No matter how much she maintained her workout schedule, Sam was losing muscle tone and mass. To make matters worse, she was finding it difficult to concentrate on one task, let alone more—a matter that was beginning to affect her life both at home and at work. When her libido all but disappeared, she came to see me.

At age fifty-three, Mel had gradually developed symptoms over approximately five years that included decreased endurance, weight gain around the waist, irritability, decreased erections, loss of morning erection, morning sluggishness, low sex drive, increased seasonal allergies, fatigue, breast enlargement, grumpiness, muscle aches and stiffness, lack of enthusiasm, and ringing in the ears. He had tried herbal remedies and found that they made his irritability worse and had no effect on any of his other symptoms. By the time he came to Signature, he had quit taking all his medications, having given up on finding a cure for his symptoms.

At age thirty-seven, Dave came to me reporting that he had been under a lot of stress for the past two years. He had recently moved to Canada from the United States, gotten married, and then had a new child. His symptoms included increased anxiety and general irritability. He found himself overreacting to the smallest issues and just unable to handle problems. He also complained of decreased endurance, weight gain around the waist, decreased erections, a "burned out" feeling, foggy thinking, memory lapses, morning sluggishness, low sex drive, fatigue, loss of sense of humor, depression, muscle aches and stiffness, lack of enthusiasm, feeling pressed for time, poor exercise tolerance, and increased caffeine consumption.

At age sixty-four, Elise had been suffering through severe menopausal symptoms for three years. Her symptoms had arisen in the wake of a hysterectomy at age sixty-one, during which she had her ovaries removed. Her periods had stopped years earlier, and she had no menopausal symptoms. However, within two months of surgery, she had severe anxiety, irritability, fatigue, severe palpitations, and chest pain. She had gone to the emergency room a number of times with severe chest pain and had undergone several cardiac workups, all of which were negative. She had foggy thinking, digestive problems, sinus problems, muscle aches and pains, and joint pain. At her first visit with me, she told me, "I get up in the morning, make my bed, and then get right back in it."

Chapter 1

THE POWER OF BIOIDENTICAL HORMONES

When Sue first came to Signature Hormones, she had a host of symptoms: hot flashes, night sweats, difficulty sleeping, and just an overall "run down" feeling. In short, her energy was gone, and she wasn't feeling like her old self. She had decreased libido—to the point that her symptoms had begun to cause problems in her relationship. She had so much difficulty concentrating that it was beginning to affect her work. And while usually a very pleasant person to be around, she found herself getting more irritable all the time, even snapping at others—family, friends, coworkers—without cause. She was struggling to multitask, making it difficult to function for a family that had always relied on her. To top it all off, she put on weight, especially around her midsection, further adding to her frustration.

One evening, while sitting with the family watching a favorite television program, a scene had her melting into tears. She completely lost control—even though she knew her reaction to the program was not normal.

Grabbing for the tissue box and apologizing between sniffles, she resolved to consult someone for help. She had heard about hormone-replacement therapy (HRT) but was skeptical of it because she'd heard it caused cancer. Then she read about bioidentical HRT and decided to give us a call.

YOUR HORMONAL SYSTEM—A TICKET INTO "THE BEST-ME CLUB"

Sue's story typifies what women in perimenopause or menopause go through daily.

Although they come to me with a feeling of isolation—believing that they alone are suffering from the problems—the truth is they're part of a much larger group of women, what we at Signature Hormones affectionately refer to as "The Best-Me Club." If you're experiencing body and mind changes that you didn't see coming, then let me be the first to welcome you to the Club.

You see, you're not alone. You're one of some twenty-five million women around the world who are experiencing the symptoms of menopause every day—from hot flashes, night sweats, and sleep disturbances to mood swings, depression, and even dementia.[1] For some women, menopause can lead to chronic and even potentially deadly conditions and diseases such as osteoporosis and cardiovascular disease.

In fact, by 2030, the World Health Organization estimates that some 1.2 billion women will be postmenopausal.[2] See what I mean when I say you're not alone?

1   K. Stephenson, P. F. Neuenschwander, and A. K. Kurdowska. "The effects of compounded bioidentical transdermal hormone therapy on hemostatic, inflammatory, immune factors; cardiovascular biomarkers; quality-of-life measures; and health outcomes in perimenopausal and postmenopausal women," *International Journal of Pharmaceutical Compounding*, 17, no. 1(Jan.-Feb. 2013):74-85, abstract accessed on U.S. National Library of Medicine National Institutes of Health, October 11, 2016, https://www.ncbi.nlm.nih.gov/pubmed/23627249.

2   Ibid.

The changes you're feeling are the result of changes in your hormonal system, a natural decline that occurs as part of the aging process.

A hormone is a chemical substance produced by the body that controls and regulates the activity of certain cells and organs. "Hormone" is derived from the Greek word *hormon*, which essentially means "urge on"—that's the role of hormones in your body.[3] They urge your cells to do specific tasks by binding to your body's receptors. I'll explain more about receptors shortly.

All your hormones are produced by the body's endocrine system, which is composed of a number of other organs and glands in your body, including these:

- adrenal glands—two thumb-sized organs located just above your kidneys

- hypothalamus—located near the base of the brain

- ovaries—part of the female reproductive system

- pancreas—part of your digestive system that helps break down food

- pituitary gland—a pea-sized gland at the base of the brain

- thyroid—a butterfly-shaped gland located low in the front of the neck

Your hormones must interact with each other through well-functioning organs in your body. For you to feel great and be healthy, your hormones must function much like a symphony orchestra—playing together and in tune. If your hormones are not balanced and playing a lovely melody, you will experience a range of symptoms.

---

3   Katharina Dalton with Wendy Holton, *Depression after Childbirth: How to Recognise, Treat, and Prevent Postnatal Illness* (Oxford: Oxford University Press, 2001).

It only takes a small amount of hormones to have a powerful effect on your body. Hormones are also very selective in their tasks, and they only work correctly in the right conditions.

Problems can arise when conditions aren't quite what those finicky hormones expect. Your hormone levels change throughout your lifetime, and many different factors can influence the amount of a particular hormone. Any change in a hormone can upset the system—too much or too little of one hormone in proportion to another can throw everything off balance.

FEAR OF TREATMENT

Unfortunately, millions of women will fail to seek out or find relief for their symptoms because of a fear of the best solution available: HRT.

HRT is a treatment for women whose hormone levels drop significantly because of menopause. It augments the body's natural hormone levels, artificially boosting hormone levels to help reduce the symptoms of menopause and help women have a better quality of life. Traditionally, HRT treatment is commonly administered as estrogen-only therapy (ET), which is for women who have had a hysterectomy and therefore enter menopause surgically, or as estrogen-with-progesterone therapy (EPT), which is for women who naturally experience menopause at midlife. However, often other hormones are also deficient and require replacement. That is why it is important to have all your hormones tested—and not just take the traditional approach of using estrogen and progesterone only.

For decades, HRT was considered a "must have" for women entering menopause. It was a go-to solution for women at the first sign of a hot flash. When I first began to practice medicine, hormones were being pushed for everything, even if a woman didn't have any symptoms. I've been in practice now since 1992, and during those first few years, I saw a lot of women who were having side effects from one of the common hormone treatments at that point, Premarin.

That sent me exploring alternatives that would help with women's symptoms and not leave them with the same side effects. It was a journey that eventually led me to offer natural or bioidentical hormones, and I've been amazed at the improvements that I've seen in patients using them.

Unfortunately, a hurdle was placed in the path of HRT progression in the early 2000s, and it has been a challenge for HRT to regain a real foothold since then.

In 2001, the findings of a long-term American study, the Women's Health Initiative (WHI), were released, and everything doctors thought they knew for twenty years was proven wrong.

The WHI was a set of clinical trials that started in 1991 and observed thousands of women who had already entered menopause and who were put on conjugated equine estrogen (CEE) and Provera to assess the effects of these drugs on them. CEE is a synthetic estrogen made from the urine of pregnant mares. Provera, also known as medroxyprogesterone acetate, is a synthetic progesterone, which is also known as a progestin. The CEE Premarin and the progestin Provera are synthetic hormones that are still widely prescribed in traditional medicine.

In the early 2000s, results of one of three WHI trials were published, five years early, because the study found an increase in breast cancer and other health risks in the women subjects who were taking CEE and Provera. Again, these were manmade (synthetic) versions of the naturally occurring hormones in a woman's body. Notably, only the subjects in the study who were taking CEE and Provera saw increased risks. Other women in the trials who were on estrogen alone, even though it was the synthetic version, did not have increased health risks.

While the WHI trials called into question the widely accepted practice of prescribing synthetic hormones in women experiencing the symptoms of perimenopause or menopause, the trials also had far more detrimental consequences—HRT itself became suspect as a treatment. Instead of pointing to the consequences related directly to the findings—that the combination of CEE and Provera raised health risks in menopausal women—the study cast doubt on the entire HRT medical field.

That doubt was amplified by the release of findings of the Million Women Study, a study based in the United Kingdom whose results were published in the UK medical journal *Lancet*. The Million Women Study looked at the history of roughly one million women, ages fifty to sixty-four, focusing primarily on their use of HRT and their incidences of breast cancer. Like the WHI trials, the Million Women Study found that women who took a synthetic estrogen along with a progestin had a substantially higher risk of breast cancer than women taking estrogen alone.

Furthermore, the American-based Heart and Estrogen/Progestin Replacement Study (HERS) found that estrogen plus progestin did nothing to prevent heart attacks or coronary heart disease, even though it reduced low-density lipoprotein (LDL)—the bad cholesterol—by 11 percent and raised high-density lipoprotein cholesterol levels (HDL)—which is the "good" cholesterol that protects against heart disease—by 10 percent.[4] Instead, the study found that HRT

---

4   "The HERS Study Results and Ongoing Studies of Women and Heart Disease,"
     National Heart, Lung, and Blood Institute, news release, August 18, 1998,
     accessed October 11, 2016, http://www.nhlbi.nih.gov/news/press-releases/1998/
     the-hers-study-results-and-ongoing-studies-of-women-and-heart-disease.

raised the risk of deep vein thrombosis and pulmonary embolism, or blood clots in the veins and lungs.

It's important to note that subjects in the Million Women Study were largely already in menopause, and those in the HERS study were postmenopausal women with known instances of heart disease who were on average sixty-seven years old.

Unfortunately for women, the results of these studies have meant that not only have the benefits of HRT been largely ignored in the years since the release of the studies' data, but that thousands of women have had to suffer through menopause and even risked death because they did not take treatment.

In fact, according to researchers from the Yale School of Medicine, almost fifty thousand unnecessary deaths occurred in the ten years following the release of the WHI findings because doctors avoided prescribing estrogen-only HRT.[5]

The Yale study pointed specifically at the WHI and HERS trials and looked at US census data and hysterectomy rates. Prior to WHI, HRT was commonly prescribed for women in surgical menopause because they had undergone a hysterectomy. More than 90 percent of women, according to the Yale study, were prescribed estrogen-only therapy to reduce their menopausal symptoms and other health risks associated with hormone deficiency. Between 2002 and 2011, according to the study, HRT declined in women ages fifty to fifty-nine.[6]

After the initial WHI damage had been done, the results of the second of three WHI trials were released. The results of that trial, which studied women with hysterectomies who were given either

---

5   Christian Nordqvist, "Withholding estrogen therapy cost tens of thousands of lives," *Medical News Today* (July 20, 2013), accessed October 11, 2016, http://www.medicalnewstoday.com/articles/263708.php.

6   Ibid.

a placebo or estrogen-only HRT, found mostly good outcomes. In fact, a later WHI study, conducted in 2011–2012, found that estrogen-only therapy over a ten-year period actually reduced instances of heart disease and breast cancer: thirteen more women per ten thousand who were not taking estrogen during that time died or developed heart disease or breast cancer.[7]

Since the WHI, Million Women, and HERS studies, there have been innumerable attempts to prove the viability of HRT one way or the other. One key to understanding these studies and deciding for yourself as to their validity is to examine the criteria each study is based on—who were the study participants, what was administered, what were the specific outcomes?

Perhaps a better way to decide whether HRT is right for you is to know exactly what happens on the inside of your body when HRT is administered.

UNDERSTANDING THE SCIENCE

Once the findings of the WHI and HERS trials were released, doctors were in a quandary, cynical of using any hormone to treat menopausal symptoms. Because the drug companies originally said the synthetic hormones were safe, and then a major study declared them unsafe, how could doctors be sure bioidentical hormones were any better?

It all comes down to understanding the science of bioidentical hormones. That goes for doctors and for you, as a potential user of HRT.

Bioidentical hormone preparations are medications containing hormones that are an exact chemical match to those made naturally by the human body.

---

7   Ibid.

Since bioidentical hormones have the same molecular structure, they more readily mimic the function of the hormones your body produces on its own, making it is easier for your body to recognize them. Your ovaries can't distinguish between your own hormones and the bioidentical ones you take as part of HRT. In hormone testing, bioidentical estradiol, the most prominent form of estrogen, is indistinguishable from your own estradiol.

The same cannot be said of the synthetic estrogen Premarin.

Premarin can't be measured because it metabolizes in the bloodstream into various other forms of estrogen that aren't detected with standard laboratory tests.

Hormone replacement works because of the action of receptor sites in the body's cells. Hormone receptors are special molecules in and on the surface of your body's cells that bind to specific hormones. Specific substances in the bloodstream "fit" specific receptor sites, and the number of receptor sites on a cell varies in accordance with nutrients and other factors in your body. When a hormone in the bloodstream "fits" a receptor site, it binds the hormones from the bloodstream to the cell, which then tells the cell to take some sort of action. Some of the actions a receptor is instructed to undertake may include the manufacture of other proteins or the replication of cells.

With this very basic understanding of how hormones work, it's always made sense to me to use all-natural compounds. If you ingest or your body absorbs something made of natural products, logically, it's better than putting something foreign in your body. For instance, if you take in a natural hormone, it will better bind to your body's receptors and function in the same way as your own hormones, whereas synthetic hormones won't behave the same way—they won't willingly bind to a cell and cause a positive action to occur.

HOW THEY'RE MADE

Bioidentical hormones are made by specialized compounding pharmacies. These pharmacies custom tailor the bioidentical formula to match each individual patient's needs.

The science of pharmaceutical compounding dates back to the origins of medicine, although it has changed over the years with the advent of mass manufacturing of drugs. Still, the goal of specially compounded formulas is to help the physician and patient achieve a more positive therapeutic outcome. While the practice of compounding medications specifically for a patient's needs is rarer these days, it is crucial for the best outcomes with HRT.

One of the common criticisms of HRT is that there is no quality oversight to the production of bioidentical hormones. Since HRT is a tremendous growth industry, there are many new players in the field of compound pharmacies. Consequently, the quality across the different pharmacies can vary tremendously, even within a single pharmacy.

The Food and Drug Administration (FDA) has stated that compound drugs "are both ethical and legal as long as they are prescribed by a licensed practitioner for a specific patient and compounded by a licensed pharmacy."[8] In Canada, where my practice is based, compounding is regulated by provincial boards of pharmacy, as stated by Health Canada, the governing body for Canada's national public health system: "Compounding must be a legitimate part of the practice of regulated healthcare professionals and must not be used as a means to bypass the federal drug review and approval system. All drug compounding and manufacturing activities performed are to be

---

8   "Compounding Answers," PCCA, accessed October 12, 2016, http://www.pccarx.com/what-is-compounding/compounding-answers.

regulated and fall under either the federal or the provincial/territorial jurisdiction."[9]

The US-based Professional Compounding Centers of America (PCCA) is one organization that has helped raise the standards in the compounding field, specifically when it comes to compounding hormones. The PCCA is a comprehensive resource for independent compound pharmacies that is registered and inspected by the FDA and the US Drug Enforcement Agency (DEA). The PCCA provides the products that the pharmacist needs to create different hormone preparations. It also developed special creams, or bases, to help administer hormones into the body, either through the skin or through a mucous membrane. The PCCA provides standards that the pharmacies that use its products must adhere to in order to promote themselves as being PCCA designated.

I rely on the PCCA because its standards are very high. Not all pharmacies belong to the PCCA, and there's no other organization that provides guidelines as reliably.

Early in my career, I discovered that not all compounding pharmacies would follow my prescription to the letter—some would alter my prescriptions based on their available supplies and without my prior approval. However, today's more stringent oversight of the industry along with my own very strict standards ensures that patients receive exactly what's been prescribed. I'm very particular about which compounding pharmacies I use for the hormones I prescribe because I have very specific instructions I need to have followed for my prescriptions.

Problems have arisen in the past if, for instance, I prescribed a 0.2 ml dosage of hormone administered from a 3 cc syringe,

9   "Policy on Manufacturing and Compounding Drug Products in Canada (POL-0051)," Health Canada, accessed October 12, 2016, http://www.hc-sc.gc.ca/dhp-mps/compli-conform/gmp-bpf/docs/pol_0051-eng.php#a7.

which amounted to two lines of cream measurable on the side of the syringe. However, if the pharmacy placed the prescription in a clicker, a pump, or a larger-size syringe, that would then alter the instructions—and the dosage—to the patient. I wouldn't find out about the change until later, after the patient had been using the cream and was not getting the anticipated results.

Today, I only work with pharmacists I've built a relationship with and who I know will precisely follow my prescription. That way, patients can administer hormones as I have specifically outlined. Some of the pharmacies I work with ship all over the world, because I've got patients both in and outside of Canada, so it's crucial that they follow my instructions to the letter.

Compounding allows me to customize your prescription based specifically on your unique needs. Based on my assessment of you when you visit my practice—which involves your medical history, sometimes a physical examination, and then lab results—I determine which hormones need to be replaced. When I review your lab tests, I determine what's normal and what's not, and how those relate to the symptoms that you have described to me. At that point, I determine what we can do to correct any hormonal deficiencies and what kind of results you should expect from your treatment.

I then write out a very specific prescription that includes which hormones I want you to receive and in what form I want you to take them. I determine the medium—cream, capsule, troche (a soft, dissolvable disk), or liquid—the dosage, and the frequency. It's a very detailed, very specific prescription. And you get one for each hormone that has been identified as being deficient and that we want to correct.

Quality compounding allows me to determine the best course of treatment by giving you the exact dosages of hormones your body needs. A compounded prescription can help you start and maintain a hormone-replacement regimen to bring your hormones back into balance. Compounding also makes it much easier to more accurately adjust the dosage, if needed, to ensure that the HRT is just right for your needs.

JULIE

Relieving Symptoms and HRT Concerns

Julie's menopause symptoms were making it hard to get through the day—they were affecting her job, her relationships, her daily life. She tried HRT from her traditional doctor but wasn't getting the relief she needed—in part because she was apprehensive about HRT in general.

While researching online for a new doctor with whom she might feel a better connection, she came across Dr. George Arnold and Signature Hormones. "I was very relieved to read about Dr. Arnold's extensive background in women's health combined with his experience with bioidentical hormone treatment," she said.

At Signature, Dr. Arnold recommended a bioidentical hormone treatment specially formulated for Julie's blood-test results, which relieved her symptoms and the concerns she had about HRT. "Under Dr. Arnold's care, I feel far more beneficial results," she said. "His gentle, professional manner and extensive knowledge of the subject helped me ten fold to deal with anxiety about the whole experience."

BENEFITS OF BIOIDENTICALS

The good news is that HRT can provide relief for your perimeno-pausal and menopausal symptoms. There are many benefits gained by the natural, customized approach of bioidentical hormone replacement therapy (BHRT), including (but not limited to):

- improved weight loss

- improved sex drive

- improved look and feel of hair and skin and nails

- improved mental health

- improved memory

- improved energy

- improved mood and emotional balance

- relief of hot flashes and night sweats

- restful and restorative sleep

- feeling yourself again

As I mentioned earlier, HRT comes in easy-to-use forms. It can be taken orally, transdermally (i.e., applied to the skin as a patch or a cream), or in some cases, administered through injection.

How the hormone is administered can impact its effect on the body. For instance, estrogen given by mouth can decrease growth hormone and increase liver enzymes, increase body inflammation leading to an increase in C-reactive protein, increase the incidence of gallstones, and increase sex-hormone-binding globulin (SHBG). It can lead to a decrease in testosterone and an increase in triglycerides, blood pressure, and weight gain. However, transdermal estrogen—estrogen given through the skin—has none of these effects and can lower body inflammation, lower triglycerides, and decrease C-reactive protein.

I will talk more about the different forms of administration in the chapters ahead. For now, suffice it to say that I will determine the best form of medication for you when you visit us at Signature Hormones. I want to ensure you that we'll treat you with the safest, most effective form of the hormone to give you the best outcomes.

EVELYN

Not One-Size-Fits-All

For Evelyn, getting relief for her menopausal symptoms was a matter of finding a practitioner who understood her individual needs. When night sweats and hot flashes set in as part of her menopausal symptoms, Evelyn sought help from her general practitioner. He recommended prescription HRT pills. But Evelyn found that the one-size-fits-all prescription not only didn't resolve her symptoms, but the pills further exacerbated her mood swings by causing a range of side effects.

A friend told Evelyn about how Signature's solutions had relieved her symptoms, so Evelyn made an appointment to see Dr. Arnold. He suggested a bioidentical HRT course of treatment, and soon Evelyn's symptoms were nearly nonexistent. "I was so pleased with my outcomes that I have since suggested other friends look into bioidenticals through Dr. Arnold," Evelyn said.

DISPELLING THE MYTHS OF
BIOIDENTICAL HORMONES

Whether you're looking at traditional or alternative forms of hormone treatment, there are different ways to approach the same problem. For instance, in Canada, where we have a national, provincial health care system, if a woman comes to me with menopausal symptoms and wants payment for her care to be covered by the government, I'm limited to prescribing traditional medication. The government recognizes Premarin and Provera for treatment of menopausal symptoms, but it doesn't cover bioidentical hormones, because it considers them to be an alternative, or complementary, treatment.

Other governing bodies are cautious in recommending bioidenticals as viable forms of treatment for menopause. The position of the FDA and The Endocrine Society is that there is little or no evidence to support claims that bioidentical hormones are safer or more effective. The Society of Obstetricians and Gynaecologists of Canada (SOGC) has also voiced concerns about BHT, saying it is composed of "custom-mixed recipes that are not regulated or approved" with "no scientific evidence of the effect they may have on the body. Currently, there are no long-term studies on bioidenticals that demonstrate their effectiveness or safety."[10]

Part of the problem with bioidenticals gaining traction is the hand that major pharmaceutical companies have in the issue. Big Pharma, as the pharmaceuticals industry is often known, can't patent naturally occurring compounds, so it won't back them.

However, I prefer bioidentical hormones purely because of the hormones themselves. I've mentioned some specific studies, but there

---

10 "Public Education Pamphlets," The Society of Obstetricians and Gynaecologists of Canada (SOGC), accessed October 12, 2016, https://sogc.org/publications-resources/public-information-pamphlets.html?id=15.

are many more that have clearly shown bioidentical hormones are safer than synthetic hormones. They're "alternative" because they're another option, a complementary treatment that is better than the synthetic hormones paid for by the government.

Over time, the awareness of natural or bioidentical hormones has increased through their promotion by well-known celebrities such as Suzanne Somers and others in the entertainment industry.

In the February 2009 edition of *O, The Oprah Magazine,* Oprah Winfrey said menopause caught her "off guard" and that she's taking bioidentical hormones that have made a big improvement in how she feels. Oprah felt "out of kilter" and for two years had "issues" that she suspected were hormonal. Upon a friend's recommendation, Winfrey went to a doctor who specializes in hormones.

Winfrey wrote that the hormone specialist told her that her "hormonal tank was empty" and gave her a prescription for bioidentical estrogen. "After one day on bioidentical estrogen, I felt the veil lift," Winfrey wrote. "After three days, the sky was bluer, my brain was no longer fuzzy, my memory was sharper. I was literally singing and had a skip in my step."

Winfrey wasn't recommending bioidentical hormones for every menopausal woman. Instead, she urged women to "take charge of your health" and said it's time to "start the conversation" about menopause and bioidentical hormones.

Many women research bioidentical hormones before coming to me. They look into their safety and benefits and what they believe may be best for them. Often, having researched traditional vis-à-vis bioidentical, they'll decide bioidentical is more appropriate for them.

Because patients who come to me have so many questions, it's part of my practice to try to clear up any misconceptions. Here are some of the common misconceptions I hear from patients, and some of my responses to their concerns:

Q: "Doctor, I read that the industry isn't regulated. Is that true?"

A: No. There are bodies around like PCCA that provide quality oversight for the production of bioidentical hormones to ensure that the pharmacists are meeting the quality standards that are expected.

Q: "My doctor is totally against bioidentical hormones."

A: Typically, this kind of attitude stems from unsupported biases because the physician making the comment has not taken the time to carefully investigate what BHT is all about.

The trouble is that many times a patient has established a relationship—sometimes over many years—with his or her family doctor. There's a bond, a trust that's been built up. The patient may know that the doctor won't necessarily be able to offer HRT but is looking for the doctor's blessing or support before proceeding.

I have patients who have been sent to me from their primary care doctors—physicians who know my reputation and that I strongly believe in the safety and efficacy of bioidentical hormones. Unfortunately, too often I also hear from my patients that they were disappointed in their family doctor's reaction when they asked about HRT. One of the biggest letdowns is when patients find out someone they thought had their best interests at heart is completely against something they had their hearts set on. "What are you doing?" the doctor may say. "Are you nuts? If you go on it, you're doing it without my approval." I would much rather hear that their doctor either didn't know enough about it to prescribe it or recommended them to someone like me, a board-certified gynecologist who knows both the traditional and the alternative side of medicine.

Q: "There is no evidence that bioidenticals are safe."

A: Several studies conducted over the years show that bioidentical hormones are both safe and efficacious. They provide treatments for menopausal and perimenopausal symptoms, and in some cases, can even help prevent or lessen the risk of disease. I'll be sharing more studies in the chapters ahead, but for now, consider the findings of studies in 2005 and 2007, which looked at a massive study by French researchers of more than one hundred thousand women over a twelve-year period. The first study, known as the E3N, was conducted by the European Prospective Investigation into Cancer and Nutrition (EPIC) and recruited women ages forty to sixty-five to look at diet and hormones in relation to environment, biology, and genetics as potential risk factors for cancer and other major chronic diseases.

- Fournier (2005): A 2005 review of more than fifty-four thousand women who were part of the renowned E3N-EPIC cohort study found that the risk for breast cancer significantly increased if synthetic progestin was combined with estrogen, but it was reduced if estrogen was combined with natural progesterone.[11]

- Fournier (2007): In 2007, another study looked at more than eighty thousand women who were followed for more than eight years as part of the E3N-EPIC study. This study also found that women who used only estrogen had a non significant increase of 1.29 times the risk for breast cancer. The study group that was administered estrogen plus a progestin saw an increased risk of breast cancer up

---

11   Agnès Fournier, Franco Berrino, and Françoise Clavel-Chapelon, "Unequal risks for breast cancer associated with different hormone replacement therapies: results from the E3N cohort study," *Breast Cancer Research and Treatment* 107, issue 1 (January 2008): 103-111, abstract accessed on U.S. National Library of Medicine National Institutes of Health, October 12, 2016, https://www.ncbi.nlm.nih.gov/pmc/articles/PMC2211383/, doi: 10.1007/s10549-007-9523-x.

to 1.69 times that of the control group. However, when progesterone was combined with estrogen, not only was the risk of breast cancer eliminated—it was actually reduced.[12]

Q: "What snake oil are you peddling now?"

A: Some people believe HRT operates essentially on a placebo effect, that bioidentical hormones are something a woman takes that she just imagines are making her feel better. Studies have clearly shown that natural hormone medications have beneficial effects in treating perimenopausal and menopausal symptoms.

Q: "I've heard they cause cancer. Is this true?"

A: Anything used in a high enough dose, from a hormone point of view, has the potential to cause cancer. At Signature, we use an estrogen product that is made up primarily of the weak estrogen, estriol, which has evidence to support its cancer-preventing qualities. Progesterone also down-regulates the number of estrogen receptors that are present in the body, decreasing the likelihood of developing cancer.

However, just as some women who aren't on any hormone therapy at all will develop cancer, some women on HRT will develop cancer that has nothing to do with the HRT they're taking. We want to make sure when using hormones that we're not increasing that risk, and that's possible because of the cancer-preventing qualities, especially with the estriol and progesterone combination.

---

12   Agnès Fournier, et. al., "Breast cancer risk in relation to different types of hormone replacement therapy in the E3N-EPIC cohort," *International Journal of Cancer* 114, no. 3 (April 2005): 448-54, abstract accessed on U.S. National Library of Medicine National Institutes of Health, October 12, 2016, https://www.ncbi.nlm.nih.gov/pubmed/15551359, doi: 10.1002/ijc.20710.

Q: "Should you really be taking a hormone replacement?"

A: Often, this is a statement made by a physician who is considering the patient's medical history. Some women also voice a similar concern: "I can't take HRT because of a family history of breast cancer." A distant family relative who's had breast cancer would not necessarily be a factor that's going to increase your risk. As the studies have shown, bioidenticals in the right combination—estriol/estradiol plus progesterone—do not increase breast-cancer risk but can actually provide some protection *against* breast cancer.

Whatever the concern, I prefer to address it with my patients up front. I want to be sure to provide the evidence to help you feel safe and comfortable with your decision to embark on the HRT journey.

ANDROPAUSE

Menopause for Men

As a menopausal woman, you may have also noticed changes in your man. That's because as men age, they also undergo hormonal changes. At Signature Hormones, we also treat men for hormonal imbalance.

Although symptoms may vary from person to person, common symptoms of andropause in a man include:

- lower sex drive
- difficulties getting erections or erections that are not as strong as usual
- lack of energy
- depression
- irritability and mood swings

- loss of strength or muscle mass

- increased body fat

- hot flashes

Often, after I've helped a woman feel better with HRT, she tells me her man can no longer keep up with her and looks to me for help with him.

Interestingly, while men will come to see us for fertility issues—HRT can help couples who are having trouble getting pregnant—they tend to be reluctant to pursue help with the same symptoms of aging as women experience. Often, however, they will pursue a solution at the urging of their female partners. Once your man sees the difference in you, he's likely to be more open to discussion.

If your man is experiencing the symptoms of andropause, let us help him at Signature Hormones.

AN HRT BELIEVER

After Sue's experience with bioidentical HRT—her symptoms were all but gone after a few months, and she was even motivated to lose twenty pounds—she became a true believer and has referred several friends to my practice.

As with all my patients, Sue's first visit started with the two of us talking about her health history. I listen to every patient to understand more about them and their symptoms, which may indicate an underlying hormone imbalance. I also want to answer any questions you have about HRT—to help you feel completely comfortable with any therapy prescribed.

Your first visit may also include a physical examination, although one is not always needed. Testing is done through saliva, urine, or blood to look at the different hormone levels to match those up with your symptoms. The lab tests are just to confirm what I suspect is going on with your situation.

From there, we put together a customized program of hormone replacement using natural hormones to address your issues. We schedule a follow-up visit to help revise your prescriptions, if needed, and to ensure that you are on track with your outcomes.

Now, let's look at the various hormones that may be causing you issues and what some of those might be. Many women experience imbalances with more than one of these hormones.

Chapter 2 Symptom Chart: *Thyroid*

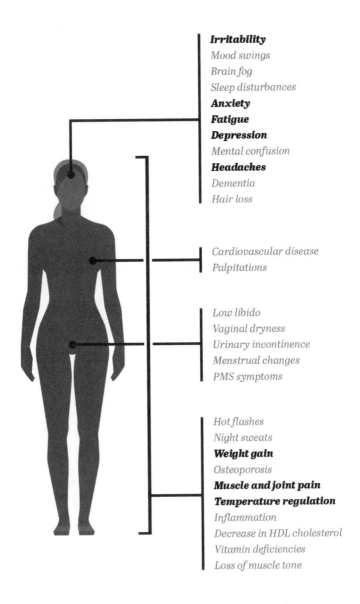

Irritability
Mood swings
Brain fog
Sleep disturbances
Anxiety
Fatigue
Depression
Mental confusion
Headaches
Dementia
Hair loss

Cardiovascular disease
Palpitations

Low libido
Vaginal dryness
Urinary incontinence
Menstrual changes
PMS symptoms

Hot flashes
Night sweats
Weight gain
Osteoporosis
Muscle and joint pain
Temperature regulation
Inflammation
Decrease in HDL cholesterol
Vitamin deficiencies
Loss of muscle tone

Chapter 2

THYROID: IT'S NOT ALL IN YOUR HEAD

One day while driving down the road, Erin suddenly felt an overwhelming sense that something was wrong. By the time she could pull over and park the car, her heart was racing—nearly pounding out of her chest—and she had broken out in a visible sweat. Eventually, she was able to calm herself, but the attack was only one of many she would begin to experience.

At age forty-eight, Erin had begun noticing changes in her body. In addition to irregular menstrual cycles, she was gaining weight despite her workouts. Over time, she noticed her nails becoming more brittle, and her hair brush seemed to come away with more strands every time she used it. She even began to lose hair in her eyebrows, and over time, she found she had to shave her legs less often. She felt the cold more and more, and her bones and joints ached—but she had written off her symptoms to a chronic cold and arthritis.

Finally, she visited me at Signature Hormones where I found Erin was suffering from the symptoms of underactive thyroid, a condition known as hypothyroidism.

HYPOTHYROIDISM: SOLVING THE MYSTERY

Hypothyroidism is a condition in which the thyroid gland doesn't produce enough thyroid hormone to keep the body operating at optimum levels. The thyroid hormone's main function is to keep the body's metabolism running at optimum efficiency. When your thyroid-hormone levels are low, your metabolism slows, which can lead to a host of other conditions.

The Thyroid Foundation of Canada estimates that some two hundred million people worldwide have some form of thyroid disease.[13] In Canada alone, it's estimated that one in ten people suffer from a thyroid condition—half of which have not been diagnosed.[14] The American Thyroid Association also estimates that women are at least five times more likely than men to have a thyroid problem and that one in eight women is likely to develop a thyroid disorder sometime in her life.[15]

You don't have to be a member of "The Best-Me Club" to suffer from low or underactive thyroid. But like menopausal symptoms, women suffering from low thyroid sometimes have trouble finding relief from their traditional doctors.

That's because hypothyroidism is a somewhat elusive condition. It can be difficult to identify a thyroid problem based on the symptoms, since its symptoms can resemble any number of *other* conditions. Take a look at some of the common signs and symptoms that I see in patients with low thyroid-hormone production and you'll see what I mean:

---

13   "About Thyroid Disease," The Thyroid Foundation of Canada, accessed October 14, 2016, http://www.thyroid.ca/thyroid_disease.php.

14   Ibid.

15   "General Information/Press Room," American Thyroid Association, accessed October 14, 2016, http://www.thyroid.org/media-main/about-hypothyroidism/.

- depression
- anxiety/panic attacks
- weight gain
- fluid retention
- constipation
- headaches/migraine headaches
- brittle, ridged, striated, thickened nails
- rough, dry skin
- menstrual irregularities
- inability to concentrate
- muscle cramps/pain and joint pain
- decreased sexual interest
- excess formation of cerumen (earwax) in the ear canal
- loss of the latter one-third of the eyebrows, known as "Queen Anne's sign" or "sign of Hertoghe"

- cold hands and feet
- low body temperature
- fatigue
- PMS
- agitation/irritability
- hair loss on the head, front and back
- hair loss in varying amounts from legs, axilla, and arms
- fibrocystic breast disease
- decreased memory
- infertility
- loss of eyelashes, or eyelashes that are not as thick
- recurrent miscarriage
- cold intolerance

The important role of thyroid hormones in the body's functions cannot be overstated. A poorly functioning thyroid can lead to many serious health issues, including cardiac disease, diabetes, lupus, arthritis, and difficulties with reproduction. However, early assessment and treatment can often reduce the severity or the onset of these diseases.[16]

---

16   "About Thyroid Disease," The Thyroid Foundation of Canada, accessed October 14, 2016, http://www. thyroid.ca/thyroid_disease.php.

UNDERACTIVE THYROID IN MEN

Low thyroid is not a women-only problem. When men experience low thyroid, the symptoms are similar to those in women and can include:

- weight gain

- hair loss

- fatigue

- dry skin

- cold intolerance

- constipation

- mood changes

Just like women, men can see their thyroid levels return to normal—and their symptoms disappear—with HRT.

THYROID CONVERSION AND TESTING

Did you know that there are four thyroid hormones that function in our bodies? T4 (thyroxine) is an inactive hormone that must convert to T3 (triiodothyronine) to be active. T2 (diiodothyronine) increases the metabolic rate of the muscles and fat tissue, and T1 (monoiodothyronine) is a lesser hormone.

In the body, a conversion process starts with T4, which converts to T3. T3 then converts to T2, and T2 converts to T1.

Of the four thyroid hormones, two are especially key in your body's cells: thyroxine and triiodothyronine. These hormones are named for the number of iodine atoms they contain: thyroxine

(T4) has four iodine atoms, whereas triiodothyronine (T3) has three iodine atoms. The majority of hormone (93 percent) produced by the thyroid gland is T4—only 7 percent of the thyroid hormone produced by the thyroid gland is T3, the active form that your body needs. T4 is inactive until it is converted into T3. Once it is in the form of T3, it can then be used by your body's cells.

Despite this, the initial testing for thyroid problems typically doesn't test for any of the four "T" hormones. The initial testing is often only for levels of what's called thyroid-stimulating hormone (TSH).

TSH is a hormone produced in the pituitary gland, which as I mentioned in the previous chapter is a pea-sized gland attached to the base of the brain. The pituitary gland regulates the amount of TSH in your body. When the pituitary gland senses changes in thyroid hormone in your bloodstream, it secretes TSH, which then travels to the thyroid gland to stimulate the production of more thyroid hormone. Without that signal from the pituitary gland, your thyroid has no way of knowing that it's time to make more hormone. As you can imagine, a malfunctioning pituitary gland—due to disease or a disorder—can wreak havoc on your body.

However, measuring the amount of TSH in the bloodstream on its own is not always reliable. As with all hormone testing, the result needs to be examined in relation to symptoms and other thyroid test results.

It's important to note that many physicians voice concern about suppressing TSH as part of thyroid-replacement therapy, believing it can cause bone loss. However, the literature does not support that concern. Among the studies that show suppressing TSH does not lead to bone loss are:

- Franklin (1992): A long-term study of forty-nine people on thyroxine treatment for an average of just under eight years found no impact on bone-mineral density.[17]

- Muller (1995): A group of fifty women studied for a mean average of eleven years found no evidence of bone loss with a daily dose of thyroxine hormone.[18]

- Baldini (2002): A study of thirty-six premenopausal and fifty-three postmenopausal women studied for a median of forty-two months found no variances in bone mineral density between those who took thyroxine and those administered a placebo.[19]

As I write this book, there is also a considerable amount of controversy as to what level of TSH warrants further investigation if TSH is the only hormone being tested, which again, is often the case, as well as what level to aim for if treatment is administered. It used to be that, in Canada, no further investigation was done unless the TSH was above 5 mIU/L (milli-international units per liter). Now most labs have changed that to 4 mIU/L. However, if treatment is started, the level of TSH aimed for is less than 1 mIU/L.

One thing is certain when it comes to TSH: The lower the amount produced by your body, the better. That sounds odd, but it's true. Think about it: Again, TSH is the hormone that signals the

17 J. A. Franklyn, et al., "Long-term thyroxine treatment and bone mineral density," *Lancet* 340, no. 8810 (July 1992):9-13, abstract accessed on U.S. National Library of Medicine National Institutes of Health, October 13, 2016, https://www.ncbi.nlm.nih.gov/pubmed/1351654.

18 C. G. Müller, et al., "Possible limited bone loss with suppressive thyroxine therapy is unlikely to have clinical relevance," *Thyroid* 5, no. 2 (April 1995):81-7, abstract accessed on U.S. National Library of Medicine National Institutes of Health, October 13, 2016, https://www.ncbi.nlm.nih.gov/pubmed/7647577.

19 M. Baldini, et al., "Treatment of benign nodular goitre with mildly suppressive doses of L-thyroxine: effects on bone mineral density and on nodule size," *Journal of Internal Medicine* 251, no. 5 (May 2002):407-14, abstract accessed on U.S. National Library of Medicine National Institutes of Health, October 13, 2016.

thyroid to produce, so higher-than-normal TSH sugge
an underactive thyroid, one that is not doing its job (
enough thyroid hormone.

Since it appears that the level of TSH is a moving target, it is
especially important to look at all thyroid levels and not rely solely
on one test result.

Ideally, the following six blood tests should be completed to
fully evaluate thyroid function.

1. TSH

2. Free T4

3. Free T3

4. rT3 (reverse T3)

5. Anti-thyroid peroxidase antibody

6. Anti-thyroglobulin antibody

Free T4

The thyroid gland makes thyroxine (T4), which plays a key role in
several of your body's functions, including metabolism. While most
of the T4 in your body binds to protein in your cells, some of your
T4 is "free," meaning it doesn't bind. The free amount of T4 in the
blood is the amount present to work on receptors. However, thyroid
receptors have a very low affinity for T4.

Often, patients display the classic symptoms of hypothyroidism (underactive thyroid gland), yet upon testing, their free T4 level
appears to be in the "normal" range—albeit on the lower end of
normal. However, just because a hormone level returns in the normal
range on a lab test does not mean your levels should be considered
"normal" or that there is nothing the matter with you. The way you

feel, I'm sure you agree, is a very important fact that is often over-looked. That's why I consider more than just lab tests—I want to know about your symptoms, and then I use both them and your lab tests to decide how to proceed with treatment.

Free T3

T3 is the active thyroid hormone in your body, yet rarely is this level measured when a patient comes to her family doc with symptoms of thyroid dysfunction. T4 is converted to T3 in the thyroid, liver, kidney, pituitary, hypothalamus, and fat tissue. The conversion of T4 to T3 is dependent on enzymes called deiodinases, which remove atoms during the conversion process that I mentioned earlier. Deiodinases are responsible for removing one iodine atom from T4 hormones to create T3 hormones.

T3 hormones have a direct effect on the mitochondria—the powerhouse part of your cells responsible for converting oxygen and nutrients into adenosine triphosphate (ATP). ATP is the molecule created by aerobic respiration, a biological process that pulls energy from glucose and food in your bloodstream. ATP is used as energy by your body's cells.

Reverse T3 (rT3)

Sometimes T4 doesn't convert to T3; instead, it may convert to reverse T3 (rT3). Reverse T3 is a hormone similar to T3 that will also bind to T3 receptors. However, rT3 has no effect on the receptor except to block the real T3 from binding to it. A test for rT3 is now available in Canada. It's important to know if you're in fact dealing with rT3, as its presence will have a bearing on your treatment. Often, in women already on T4 replacement, treating rT3 involves decreasing the amount of T4 being given and increasing the amount of T3.

Elevated rT3 can be caused by chronic-fatigue syndrome (CFS), fibromyalgia, yo-yo dieting, heavy metal toxicity, infections, and physical and mental stressors.

Thyroid antibodies (anti-thyroid peroxidase antibody and anti-thyroglobulin antibody)

The presence of these in a blood test can indicate a gut disorder, often a gluten sensitivity. Eliminating gluten from the diet (not an easy or inexpensive undertaking), along with the use of a good probiotic, can reduce the production of thyroid antibodies and increase the ability of the gut to absorb the thyroid-hormone medication being taken. If your antibodies are high, they will interfere with the ability of your own thyroid hormone to attach to your body's thyroid receptors and will also act to break down your own thyroid hormone.

Again, it is important to remember that normal ranges on blood tests are guides only. In fact, it's common for me to see patients who have symptoms of low thyroid but whose lab tests return with values showing in the lower part of the "normal" range. By following what I know about thyroid, I administer hormone treatment, after which their levels change to the upper part of the "normal" range. More importantly, their symptoms resolve.

That's why I feel it's so important to talk to you about your symptoms and then to look at lab results in the context of what symptoms you are experiencing. If you are having symptoms, never let your doctor tell you there's nothing wrong with you just because your lab tests are "normal." HRT can return your "normal" to the upper end of the range where you will feel the difference.

CONVERSION DISRUPTORS

Hormone imbalances can be caused by a variety of factors that can disrupt the process of the inactive hormone T4 converting to the active hormone T3 that your body's cells need. For instance, several things can down-regulate deiodinases, the enzymes responsible for converting T4 to T3.

Here are some of the more common conversion disruptors.

Selenium deficiencies

Selenium is essential for human nutrition and plays a critical role in reproduction, thyroid-hormone metabolism, DNA synthesis, and protection of the cells from oxidative damage and infection.[20]

Iodine deficiency

A diet that lacks sufficient iodine can lead to an inability to adequately synthesize thyroid hormone no matter how urgent the message from the pituitary gland.

Vitamin and mineral deficiencies

Maintaining appropriate levels of zinc, iron, and vitamins A, B2, B3, B6, and C is crucial to proper hormone production and absorption.

Elevated cortisol levels

Cortisol is often called the "stress hormone" because it is released when a person is stressed. Cortisol is a steroid hormone made in the adrenal glands, but secretion of cortisol is controlled by the hypothalamus (in the brain) along with the pituitary and adrenal glands. The three of these acting together form what's known as the hypo-

---

20   "Selenium," National Institutes of Health, Office of Dietary Supplements, accessed October 13, 2016, https://ods.od.nih.gov/factsheets/Selenium-HealthProfessional/.

thalamic-pituitary-adrenal axis. Since most cells in the body have cortisol receptors, cortisol affects functions such as blood sugar levels, blood pressure, metabolism, inflammation, and memory. In women, cortisol also supports the developing fetus during pregnancy.

Diet imbalances

A diet with balanced levels of protein, carbohydrates, fats, and other foods is key to the T4-to-T3-conversion process.

For instance, a diet that lacks adequate amounts of protein can disrupt conversion. Much has been written about the amount of protein a woman should consume in menopause, as you no doubt know as a member of "The Best-Me Club." Several studies suggest thirty to forty grams of protein at each meal, and one study, conducted in 2011 by the University of Illinois, found that adding protein throughout the day can keep hunger pangs at bay while helping maintain more proportionate body composition in post-menopausal women.[21]

Very high or very low carbohydrate diets can also disrupt the conversion. It may surprise you to know that extremely low-carb diets aren't necessary for a menopausal woman to lose weight and can in fact induce depression and anxiety. However, a moderately low-carb diet—one hundred to one hundred fifty grams of carbs daily—can effectively induce weight loss or prevent weight gain while stabilizing blood sugar.[22]

Another surprise when it comes to diet: Low-fat diets, starvation diets, eating too many cruciferous vegetables, excessive alcohol use, and consuming walnuts or soy are also dietary disrupters.

---

21 "Eating protein throughout the day preserves muscle and physical function in dieting postmenopausal women, study suggests," *Science Daily* (August 11, 2011), news release, accessed October 13, 2016, https://www.sciencedaily.com/releases/2011/08/110810153710.htm.

22 Andrea Cespedes, "About Low-Carb Diet & Menopause," Livestrong.com (July 20, 2016), accessed October 13, 2016, http://www.livestrong.com/article/58925-low-carb-diet-menopause/.

Chronic illness

Conditions that cause chronic pain or fatigue and diseases that cause inflammation and autoimmunity can suppress deiodinases and impact the conversion process.

Cadmium, mercury, or lead toxicity

Exposure to toxins in the environment and in everyday life can disrupt hormones in the body and disrupt T4 to T3 conversion. From your plastic water bottle to your hand lotion to pesticides sprayed on the food you eat, toxic chemicals—hormone disruptors—pervade our modern world.

Decreased kidney or liver function

Although the thyroid and pituitary control the thyroid-hormone signals, the actual conversion of T4 to T3 happens in the kidneys and liver. When these organs are not operating at peak efficiency, the conversion is impacted, and it will manifest in the form of tiredness, weight gain, dry skin, thinning hair, and other symptoms.

Medications

Some medications can also affect the conversion of T4 to T3, including:

- Beta blockers. Typically taken to treat high blood pressure or hypertension

- Propranolol. Often prescribed for palpitations and anxiety

- Birth control pills. Control hormones

- Lithium. A mood stabilizer

- Phenytoin. To treat and prevent seizures

- Theophylline. For asthma, emphysema, and chronic bronchitis

- Chemotherapy. A treatment for some stages of cancer

TREATMENT FOR LOW THYROID

Since T4 has little effect in your body and must be converted to T3 to be used by the cells in your body, it seems a little odd that the traditional approach to treatment is to administer T4 and rely on your body to do the rest of the work. However, since the receptors for thyroid hormone in your cells have only a 10 percent affinity for T4 versus a 90 percent affinity for T3, it's important that T3 also be administered when treating an underactive thyroid.

A medication known simply as *thyroid*, which combines both T4 and T3, is readily available by prescription in Canada. In the United States, the same medication is known as Armour or desiccated thyroid. Thyroid medication can also be compounded specifically for your individual requirements.

Thyroid medication is somewhat finicky to use. Ideally, to be most effective, your thyroid medication should be taken on an empty stomach—and that means no food for one hour before or after you take it. I usually advise my patients to take their thyroid with a glass of water first thing upon waking, and then consume nothing else by mouth for one hour afterward. That includes taking no other medication, including vitamins, and especially calcium, which interferes with the absorption of thyroid replacement.

I also caution my patients about potential side effects of taking thyroid, as I do with all new medications. Too much thyroid medication can make you feel pretty lousy. It can cause you to feel "wired," giving you heart palpitations and tremors, such as shaky hands, and it can cause you to have hot flashes or a warm sensation. If any of these side effects are going to occur, they typically do so shortly after starting the medication for the first time, in which case patients are instructed to discontinue the medication and call me.

The potential for side effects is one primary reason why it's so important to start with a low dose and then gradually increase it. To ensure we're on target with the dosage, I follow you at specific intervals to test your thyroid levels and talk with you about your symptoms. Most of my patients see improvement within a week or so of taking thyroid.

I also insist on follow-up lab testing and a follow-up visit to ensure that your dosage is optimal and that you're getting the relief you need and expect.

Outside of thyroid HRT, the following can also improve thyroid function by increasing the conversion of T4 to T3:

- **Selenium.** Several studies have found selenium supplementation to be beneficial in treating autoimmune thyroid conditions.[23] Deiodinase enzymes also depend on selenium, making it essential for the T4-to-T3-conversion process.

- **Potassium.** Potassium increases the response of your body's cells to the active thyroid hormone T3. Foods high in potassium, such as bananas and potatoes, can restore low potassium levels in many cases.

- **Iodine**. Iodine is essential for production of thyroid hormone. Iodized salt is effective in preventing a deficiency in iodine.

---

23 Roland Gärtner, et al., "Selenium Supplementation in Patients with Autoimmune Thyroiditis Decreases Thyroid Peroxidase Antibodies Concentrations," *The Journal of Clinical Endocrinology & Metabolism* 87, issue 4 (January 2009), accessed October 14, 2016, http://press.endocrine.org/doi/full/10.1210/jcem.87.4.8421.

- **Iron**. Iron supplementation improves the beneficial effects of iodine.[24] Iron deficiency reduces activity by the enzyme thyroid peroxidase, which hinders the manufacturing of thyroid hormone. In one study, anemic patients who were hypothyroid and iron deficient saw improvements when treated with levothyroxine.[25]

- **Zinc**. In one study, patients with low levels of free T3, normal T4, elevated rT3, and moderate zinc deficiency saw their serum total T3, total free T3, and TSH levels normalize. They also saw their rT3 levels lower after taking zinc supplements for one year.[26] Note that it's advisable to take a copper supplement when taking zinc, as high doses of zinc can ultimately lead to a deficiency of copper.

- **Ashwagandha**. Also known as Indian ginseng or winter cherry, ashwagandha (withania somnifera) has been used for centuries to soothe mental and physical stress.[27] A study of the effects of ashwagandha extract on bipolar disorder found that an eight-week regimen of 500 mg daily decreased TSH, indicating improvements in thyroid

24 M. Zimmermann and J. Köhrle, "The impact of iron and selenium deficiencies on iodine and thyroid metabolism: biochemistry and relevance to public health," *Thyroid* 12, no. 10 (October 2002): 867-78, abstract accessed on U.S. National Library of Medicine National Institutes of Health, October 16, 2016, https://www.ncbi.nlm.nih.gov/pubmed/12487769.

25 Hakan Cinemre, et al., "Hematologic effects of levothyroxine in iron-deficient subclinical hypothyroid patients: a randomized, double-blind, controlled study," *The Journal of Clinical Endocrinology & Metabolism* 94, issue 1 (January 2009): accessed October 16, 2016, http://press.endocrine.org/doi/10.1210/jc.2008-1440?url_ver=Z39.88-2003&rfr_id=ori:rid:crossref.org&rfr_dat=cr_pub%3dpubmed.

26 S. Nishiyama, et al., "Zinc supplementation alters thyroid hormone metabolism in disabled patients with zinc deficiency," *Journal of the American College of Nutrition* 13, no. 1 (February 1994): 62-7, abstract accessed on U.S. National Library of Medicine National Institutes of Health, https://www.ncbi.nlm.nih.gov/pubmed/8157857.

27 J. M. Gannon, P. E. Forrest, and K. N. Chengappa, "Subtle changes in thyroid indices during a placebo-controlled study of an extract of Withani somnifera in persons with bipolar disorder," *Journal of Ayurveda and Integrative Medicine* 5, no. 4 (October-December 2014): 241-245, abstract accessed on U.S. National Library of Medicine National Institutes of Health, October 16, 2016, https://www.ncbi.nlm.nih.gov/pubmed/25624699.

function along with an increase of up to 24 percent in T4 levels.[28]

REBECCA

Getting Her Life Back

In her early sixties, Rebecca had begun to experience such severe night sweats that she found herself having to shower every morning and change her bedding daily. Her sleep was also severely disrupted. She found herself waking every two hours and during the day was so sleepy that she nodded off while driving along the highway. In addition, she was moody, chronically constipated, gaining weight, and had barely enough energy to get through the day. "I was so lethargic. I had no energy to do even day-to-day chores," Rebecca said. "I lost interest in seeing friends or doing extracurricular activities. And I ended up leaving my job because the lack of sleep made it too hard to cope during the day."

After failing to get relief from her primary care doctor, a friend referred Rebecca to Signature Hormones. "I don't like taking medication, but I desperately wanted my life back," Rebecca said. "Dr. Arnold helped me understand the value of hormone-replacement therapy, and I've had no adverse side effects from the thyroid pills he has placed me on."

Happily, Rebecca's life is back on track. "I have my energy back, I am sleeping through the night, and I lead a fuller life now," she said. "I was too young to stay home and miss out

---

28   Ibid.

on life due to menopause. I was extremely happy to find Dr. Arnold."

ADRENAL FATIGUE

When replacing thyroid hormone, it is important to ensure that the adrenal gland is functioning well, because the condition known as adrenal fatigue can interfere with thyroid function.

Your adrenal glands are two thumb-sized organs located just above your kidneys. As part of the endocrine system, the adrenal glands are involved in producing more than fifty hormones that operate in the body. Many of the hormones produced by the adrenal glands are essential for life, and it's their role to help keep these hormones in balance. Hormones released by the adrenal glands help regulate your metabolism, your immune system, your blood pressure, and your response to stress.

The adrenal medulla, which is the inner part of the adrenal gland, secretes the hormones epinephrine (adrenaline) and norepinephrine (noradrenaline) when you encounter an emotionally or physically stressful situation and your body needs additional energy to deal with it. That release of hormones helps you react to the perceived threat by rushing blood to your brain, heart, and muscles—what's known as the fight-or-flight response. Adrenal fatigue occurs when your adrenal glands can't keep up with the amount of stress you're experiencing.

If your adrenal function has not been evaluated—and often a family doc will not do this—a feeling of more fatigue when you either start on thyroid replacement or when your dosage is increased can be indicative of either adrenal fatigue or over-dosage of thyroid replacement.

Low magnesium levels may also interfere with your ability to tolerate thyroid replacement. You are more likely to get a racing heart or irregular heartbeats (palpitations) if your magnesium level is low. As already mentioned, you need a healthy gut to absorb thyroid medication well.

It is quite common to see thyroid dysfunction at the time of menopause, and that is why all the women I see are fully tested for thyroid function as well.

THYROID AND PREGNANCY

It has now become much more common to measure thyroid-hormone levels in women unable to conceive or those with recurrent miscarriages. It appears that optimal thyroid levels are needed for conception, and it's especially important to have optimized thyroid levels for a pregnancy to proceed normally. That's why a doctor checks the thyroid levels of women who are on thyroid medication while pregnant. It is not uncommon for the dose to need to be increased as the pregnancy progresses.

Similarly, a woman started on thyroid-hormone replacement, either prior to becoming pregnant or during the early part of her pregnancy, should continue with the medication during the six weeks following delivery. At that time, her levels should be checked to determine whether the dose should be continued, decreased, or stopped.

It is also not uncommon to develop hypothyroidism (underactive thyroid) during the postpartum period. If the symptoms that I mentioned at the beginning of this chapter are evident—depression, anxiety/panic attacks, headaches/migraines, or others—thyroid-replacement therapy may need to be started. If you see these symptoms in someone you know, please recommend that they be seen by a physician experienced in HRT.

HYPERTHYROIDISM: OVERDOING IT

Just as your thyroid gland can under-produce thyroid hormone (hypothyroidism), it can also over-produce it. Although rarer, over-production of thyroid is a condition known as hyperthyroidism.

An overproduction of thyroid hormone will cause your body's metabolism to rev up significantly and can lead to sudden weight loss (not a bad thing, you may think, but you really don't want to lose weight this way), a fast or irregular heart rate (palpitations), sweating, nervousness, and irritability. Often, you won't be able to sleep much at all and just have an extremely "wired" feeling.

If you're experiencing the symptoms of hyperthyroidism, get medical attention right away. If your doctor is not available to see you on an urgent basis, then the symptoms certainly warrant a trip to the emergency department. Lab testing, and often diagnostic imaging, will be performed to diagnose the condition.

Treatment can very quickly reduce the levels of thyroid hormone and eliminate most or all of your symptoms. Permanent treatment will sometimes involve surgery or treatment with radioactive iodine, which is quickly absorbed by the thyroid gland. It is also possible that, following treatment, you may go from being hyperthyroid to being hypothyroid. That's why it is important to see a doctor who treats both underactive and overactive thyroid disorders to ensure that you are getting the best treatment for *you*.

DISPELLING THE MYTHS OF THYROID-REPLACEMENT THERAPY

Here are some of the misconceptions I hear from patients about thyroid-replacement therapy.

Q: "I won't have to be on HRT for thyroid forever, will I?"
A: For most patients, the inability of your thyroid gland to produce your needed amount of thyroid hormone does not improve with either treatment or with time. In other words, replacement is typically required on an ongoing basis.

Q: "If I go on HRT, won't it make my own thyroid production worse?"
A: Taking thyroid hormone will not lead to a faster decline of your own thyroid production.

Q: "Doesn't thyroid-replacement therapy cause cancer?"
A: There are no cancer-causing effects related to thyroid medication. In patients with thyroid cancer who have had their thyroid gland removed, taking thyroid medication is absolutely required for the body to function normally.

YOU KNOW YOU

Nobody knows your body better than you do. When Erin's health began to decline, she knew something was wrong, but she just wasn't sure what. That took a visit to Signature, where we put her on thyroid-replacement therapy.

Today, Erin's symptoms are in check, as are her anxiety attacks—no more getting waylaid on the way to her destination.

If you have symptoms and signs of an underactive thyroid (hypothyroidism), please get yourself checked. If your traditional doctor tells you "it's all in your head," don't be dissuaded—you may be hypothyroid, not paranoid. Pursue relief from a doctor who will look at the big picture—someone who will listen to your symptoms and undertake a full lab investigation.

Remember: When it comes to laboratory tests, "normal" doesn't necessarily mean there is nothing wrong—especially when your symptoms tell you otherwise. The symptoms of hypothyroidism do not disappear on their own. In fact, they typically worsen with time. With treatment, you'll find yourself symptom-free in no time.

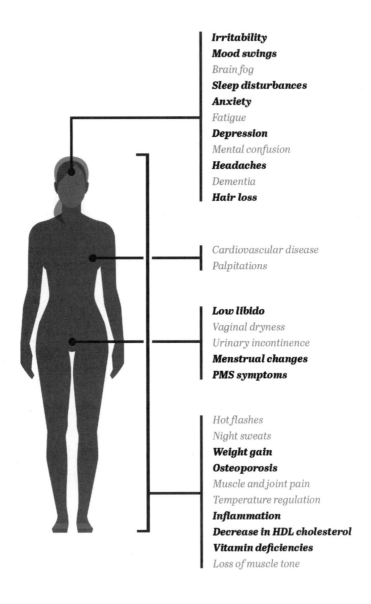

Irritability
Mood swings
Brain fog
Sleep disturbances
Anxiety
Fatigue
Depression
Mental confusion
Headaches
Dementia
Hair loss

Cardiovascular disease
Palpitations

Low libido
Vaginal dryness
Urinary incontinence
Menstrual changes
PMS symptoms

Hot flashes
Night sweats
Weight gain
Osteoporosis
Muscle and joint pain
Temperature regulation
Inflammation
Decrease in HDL cholesterol
Vitamin deficiencies
Loss of muscle tone

PROGESTERONE: THE FIRST HORMONE TO DECLINE

Alongside her declining energy levels, Jane, age forty-seven, found herself increasingly depressed and feeling anxious about everyday things that were likely not to be a problem—bills coming due, meeting deadlines, the car breaking down. She was having trouble with her sex drive—to the frustration of both her and her husband—and she was beginning to lose sleep. Her menstrual cycle had begun to be sporadic, causing her further frustration.

She came to me with her symptoms, and after talking with her and performing lab tests, I diagnosed her as being perimenopausal with a low level of free testosterone, a very low level of progesterone, a relatively normal level of the estrogen estradiol, and a moderately elevated level of follicle-stimulating hormone (FSH) that was not yet in the menopausal range. FSH is a hormone released by the pituitary gland that helps manage the menstrual cycle and stimulates the ovaries to produce eggs.

I started her on a progesterone cream twice a day, and within weeks, Jane saw her symptoms turn around.

THE ROLE OF PROGESTERONE

One reason for the increase in perimenopausal and menopausal symptoms is the decline in progesterone, which is typically the first hormone to start declining in a woman's body. Progesterone is produced naturally by the body until you reach your mid- to late thirties, at which point production begins to decline. Along with that decline, you'll begin to experience subtle changes in your periods, your moods, and your level of comfort with your own body. Progesterone continues to be made in the ovaries until you enter menopause. After menopause, a small amount of progesterone continues to be made in the adrenal glands.

Progesterone is the main female reproductive system hormone. Progesterone prepares the inner lining of the uterus for pregnancy by signaling for its walls to thicken in preparation for accepting a fertilized egg. Progesterone also keeps the uterus's muscles from contracting so that it doesn't reject the egg, and the production of progesterone also prevents ovulation. When a pregnancy does not occur, progesterone levels lower, the glandular structure in the ovary known as the *corpus luteum* breaks down, and menstruation occurs. If conception occurs, progesterone production helps support the growing fetus. I'll discuss this more in the next chapter.

Common signs and symptoms of low progesterone include:

- anxiety
- depression
- irritability
- mood swings
- insomnia (trouble sleeping)
- pain and inflammation
- nervousness
- use of antidepressants
- weight gain
- decreased sex drive
- decreased HDL cholesterol
- stress

- excessive bleeding with periods (menorrhagia)
- osteoporosis

- migraine headaches right before your period
- deficiency of zinc and vitamins A, B6, and C

Declining progesterone can be addressed with HRT. Adding a little progesterone back in can reverse some of the aforementioned symptoms.

PROGESTERONE VERSUS PROGESTIN

Earlier, I discussed the controversy over natural progesterone versus synthetic progestin in HRT.

As I mentioned, Provera, which is still widely prescribed, is not a natural progesterone. It is a progestin, which is a synthetic version of progesterone.

Progestins do not produce the same effects as natural progesterone. Progestins, such as Provera, can cause increased appetite and fluid retention, leading to weight gain. They can make you irritable and depressed, lower your energy, give you headaches, and cause breast tenderness.

Worse, progestins can interfere with your own body's production of progesterone and can intensify the symptoms of low progesterone. Progestins do not help balance the all-important hormone estrogen. In fact, progestins counteract many of the positive effects that estrogen has on serotonin, a mood-enhancing neurotransmitter in your brain. Neurotransmitters are the body's chemical messengers responsible for sending signals that tell your organs how to function. Progestins stop the protective effects that estrogen has on your heart and can even cause spasms of your coronary arteries. Progestins increase your LDL cholesterol (the bad stuff) and decrease HDL cholesterol (the good stuff).

The only good that comes from taking progestins is protection of your uterus.

On the other hand, natural progesterone has all the following positive effects. These effects are not experienced with a synthetic progesterone like Provera:

- helps balance estrogen
- leaves the body quickly
- improves sleep (especially if given orally)
- has a calming effect
- lowers high blood pressure
- helps the body use and eliminate fats
- lowers cholesterol
- may protect against breast cancer
- increases your metabolic rate
- acts as a natural diuretic
- acts as a natural antidepressant
- is anti-inflammatory
- protects the nervous system
- enhances the action of thyroid hormones
- improves libido
- stimulates the formation of new bone

With everything that natural progesterone has to offer, why would you ever use a synthetic progesterone?

MARY O

A Happy Patient, A Happy Family

Mary couldn't believe the changes her body underwent in the span of a few years. In addition to brain fog, muscle and joint pain, and lack of energy, her skin had become extremely dry and her hair had lost its sheen. Her libido had disappeared and she'd become moody. And in only five years, she'd gained sixty pounds without a significant change in her diet or activity level. "My life stopped," she said. "I had no energy for friends or family, the latter of which put a great strain on my home life. I was in pain all the time, and the weight gain added to my depression. I was aging rapidly—and not gracefully."

Mary decided to consult with Dr. George Arnold at Signature Hormones because she was "getting nowhere fast" with her family doctor. "His answer to my symptoms was to eat less and move more. But the less food I took in, the more weight I gained," she said. "I was so frustrated. How did a woman who was active, fit, and social end up with my symptoms?"

She had read about bioidentical hormones online, so when Dr. Arnold prescribed progesterone to resolve her problems with estrogen dominance and underactive thyroid, she readily agreed to try the treatment. Her pains disappeared, her muscles gained back some of their strength, her hair texture improved, and her skin is softer and glows. Plus, her energy returned, and she lost more than half the weight she had gained—without even trying. "I'm social again," Mary said. "I'm happy, but best of all, my family is happy!"

Admittedly, it took more than a year on hormone therapy for Mary to get her life back fully. But overall, she said, her experience with Dr. Arnold and Signature has been positive. "He always listens and never rushes me," she said. "He always answers my questions and addresses my concerns and suggestions."

PROGESTERONE AND BREAST CANCER

Progesterone receptors are found in the heart, brain, breasts, blood vessels, kidneys, and uterus. There are three subclasses of progesterone receptors—PRA, PRB, PRC—and each have different cellular activities. For instance, the ratio of PRA-to-PRB is approximately 1-to-1 in normal human breast tissue. Synthetic progestins alter the ratio, which may be an indicator of how progestins increase breast-cancer risk.

As I mentioned in chapter 1, the Women's Health Initiative trial found a link between synthetic hormones and breast cancer, with the main cause of the increase in breast cancer not due to Premarin (synthetic estrogen) but to Provera (a progestin or synthetic progesterone). Since then, numerous studies, including the French E3N-EPIC cohort study also mentioned in chapter 1, have consistently shown a decreased risk for breast cancer when natural progesterone levels are adequate, and some have found that HRT with bioidenticals not only doesn't cause cancer, but it can actually reduce the instances of breast cancer.

- Cowan (1981): One study that, for thirteen to thirty-three years, prospectively followed 1,083 women treated for infertility found the premenopausal risk for breast cancer to be 5.4 times higher in women with low progesterone levels. There were ten times as many deaths from breast cancer in the low progesterone group compared with those with normal progesterone levels.[29] The high-progesterone group in the study actually had more risk factors for breast cancer, highlighting the importance of that parameter.

---

29   L. D. Cowan, et al. "Breast cancer incidence in women with a history of progesterone deficiency," *American Journal of Epidemiology*, 114, no. 2 (1981): 209-217, abstract accessed on U.S. National Library of Medicine National Institutes of Health, October 12, 2016, https://www.ncbi.nlm.nih.gov/pubmed/7304556.

- Badwe (1994)[30], Mohr (1996)[31]: These studies found that women with low progesterone have significantly worse breast-cancer survival rates than those with more optimal progesterone levels.

- Ross, et. al. (2000): Combined estrogen and synthetic progestin increased the risk of breast cancer by approximately 25 percent for each five years of use compared to estrogen alone.[32]

- Chang (1995): This double-blind, placebo-controlled study examined the effects of estrogen and progesterone on women prior to surgery for removal of a lump in the breast. Patients were given placebo, estrogen, transdermal progesterone, or both estrogen and transdermal progesterone for ten to thirteen days before breast surgery. Progesterone decreased breast-cancer-cell proliferation rates by 400 percent, while estrogen increased cell proliferation rates by 230 percent. Progesterone plus estradiol inhibited the estrogen-induced breast-cell proliferation.[33]

These studies represent just a sampling of the findings over the years that show the benefits of progesterone in protecting against breast cancer.

---

30 R. A. Badwe, et al., "Serum progesterone at the time of surgery and survival in women with premenopausal operable breast cancer," *European Journal of Cancer* 30A, no. 4 (1994): 445–448, abstract accessed on U.S. National Library of Medicine National Institutes of Health, October 16, 2016, https://www.ncbi.nlm.nih.gov/pubmed/8018400.

31 P. E. Mohr, et al., "Serum progesterone and prognosis in operable breast cancer," *British Journal of Cancer* 73, no. 12 (1996): 1552–1555, abstract accessed on U.S. National Library of Medicine National Institutes of Health, October 16, 2016, https://www.ncbi.nlm.nih.gov/pubmed/8664128.

32 Ronald K. Ross, et al., "Effect of Hormone Replacement Therapy on Breast Cancer Risk: Estrogen Versus Estrogen Plus Progestin," *Journal of the National Cancer Institute* 92, no. 4 (2000): 328–332, accessed October 16, 2016, http://jnci.oxfordjournals.org/content/92/4/328.full.

33 K. J. Chang, et al., "Influences of percutaneous administration of estradiol and progesterone on human breast epithelial cell cycle in vivo," *Fertility and Sterility* 63, no. 4 (1995): 785–791, abstract accessed on U.S. National Library of Medicine National Institutes of Health, October 16, 2016, https://www.ncbi.nlm.nih.gov/pubmed/7890063.

PERIMENOPAUSE: RECOGNIZING THE SIGNS

Perimenopause is a time of transition leading up to menopause. During perimenopause, your hormones are starting to change, and along with that change, symptoms start to appear. During this natural transition, the body undergoes biologic changes resulting from declining ovarian hormone production. Perimenopause can last four to six years (sometimes longer) and usually ends after twelve months of amenorrhea (no period), which is when menopause kicks in.

It is not at all uncommon for this transition time to start as early as the mid-thirties. You may find that you, or more likely those around you, notice your mood changing. It is common for those mood changes to be more noticeable in the seven to ten days leading up to your period. During that time, your breasts may be sore, and you may find that you are not sleeping quite as well—you may even have some hot flashes and night sweats. You may start to notice some cycle and period changes with your menstrual bleeding getting heavier and lasting longer, and the number of days from the start of one period to the next starting to decrease.

Other signs and symptoms that can indicate perimenopause include joint pain or bloating. Perhaps depression has become a problem. You may be so busy juggling a household and a career that you are quick to shrug off decreased sex drive, memory lapses, lack of focus, lack of concentration, and difficulty with multitasking—all things you were once able to do effortlessly—as just a matter of "getting older" or just part of being under a lot of stress. But these are all symptoms of perimenopausal hormone change. Often my patients complain of foggy thinking, unexplainable weight gain, and occasionally more severe symptoms, such as panic attacks, starting during perimenopause. Many say they just are not as productive as they were or want to be.

It is very common to feel like you are the only one experiencing these symptoms. But that's not at all the case—in fact, in my practice, we consider perimenopause to be the first step toward entry into "The Best-Me Club."

Many women whom I see often find real solace in discussing their concerns and symptoms with friends, which helps them realize that they are not alone in this journey. They also often realize that there is treatment that can be used safely that will correct and either reduce or eliminate their symptoms.

As I said, it is the people closest to you—your coworkers, partners, kids—who first notice changes in your declining mood. Fortunately, they're also the first to notice improvement when it occurs following treatment. If others are commenting on changes in you, it is probably time to take note and investigate what might be causing your symptoms.

Unfortunately, as with many midlife symptoms, it is very common for women I see to have been treated by their own docs for some of the problems they're reporting. The most common story I hear is that they've been to the doctor for depression and been prescribed an antidepressant. However, since the cause of their depression was never identified, only the symptoms of the depression have been treated.

Whatever the symptom, it's a great disservice to treat only it and not the cause of it, and doing so minimizes the optimal result that is available to you. The best way to resolve symptoms is to treat the cause.

NATURAL MENOPAUSE

Menopause is divided into two different categories: surgical menopause and natural menopause. Surgical menopause occurs when both ovaries are removed from women still having periods. Typically, when a woman's ovaries are surgically removed, she immediately enters menopause.

Natural menopause is a condition that every healthy woman experiences when she reaches middle age, typically between the ages of thirty-five and fifty-nine, with age fifty-one being average. The duration of menopause varies for every woman but normally lasts several years and transverses a course that is impossible to predict. From a clinical point of view, you are considered menopausal once you have gone for an entire year without a period.

In menopause, the ovaries produce less estrogen and progesterone. Natural menopause occurs when your ovaries run out of eggs. When that happens, there is an increase in FSH (follicle-stimulating hormone) from your pituitary gland. FSH tries to get your ovaries to develop eggs, but since there aren't any eggs there to develop, nothing happens. FSH is the hormone that is typically measured to determine whether a woman is menopausal.

The earlier you become menopausal, the worse the symptoms tend to be. It remains a mystery as to why some women seem to stop their periods and have no symptoms at all and others are incapacitated when their periods stop. I suspect that in the women who have no symptoms there is still a small amount of hormone being produced. In fact, a patient of mine, Liz, was in her sixties when she ended up having a hysterectomy and her ovaries removed. Although her menstrual cycle had stopped years earlier, she had no menopausal symptoms at all. After she had the hysterectomy, she developed classic symptoms of menopause for the first time.

Interestingly, for years, gynecologists were taught to advise any woman age forty-five or older who was having a hysterectomy to also consider having her ovaries removed. By having both procedures done at once, it was believed she had a better chance of preventing ovarian cancer from occurring. Instead, it has been proven that removing ovaries likely causes far more harm—osteoporosis occurs sooner, hip fractures occur at a younger age—and it does not reduce the incidence of ovarian cancer. In fact, studies have shown that there remains some function as far as the ovaries producing hormones in some women into their late seventies and early eighties. If your ovaries are healthy, leave them inside where they belong. Do not consent to have your healthy ovaries removed.

PERIMENOPAUSE AND MENOPAUSE SYMPTOMS

The symptoms you may experience when going through perimenopause and menopause vary. The symptoms of menopause are similar to those of perimenopause, they just tend to be far worse and more consistent. HRT with bioidentical hormones can reduce or eliminate most or all of these symptoms.

Hot flashes are a very common symptom for women entering and in menopause caused by the ovaries decreasing their production of the hormone estrogen. Hot flashes can occur at any time and may produce flushed red skin. A hot flash occurs when the small blood vessels in your skin suddenly dilate and you get a rush of body temperature (think hot) blood suddenly coming to your skin.

Night sweats are usually more intense than hot flashes. Severity of night sweats varies, but they can also be accompanied by chills, nausea, headaches, and even an irregular heartbeat. These symptoms can easily disrupt sleep patterns.

Irritability/mood swings are a result of an intense imbalance of hormones greatly affecting the level of serotonin in the brain, which is responsible for the stability of emotions.

Loss of libido is the decrease in the desire to be sexually active. The drop in the hormones estrogen, progesterone, and testosterone is responsible for lower energy and decreased sex drive. Arousal and orgasm are still possible, but the hormonal imbalance occurring in menopause can further exacerbate the lack of sexual desire and even cause a psychological impact.

Vaginal dryness is the result of vaginal walls thinning as estrogen declines, leading to less lubrication and elasticity, resulting in irritation and itching and even pain during intercourse.

Irregular heartbeat is the result of fluctuating hormone levels, which correlate to cortisol levels and to fluctuating blood pressure, which affects the vasodilatation (widening) of the arteries and the autonomous nervous system that regulates the heartbeat. Irregular heartbeat can lead to fatigue and anxiety.

Urinary urgency/incontinence is the inability to keep urine in the bladder during sneezing, laughing, or coughing. As estrogen decreases during menopause, so does control of the bladder, since this hormone helps with the strength of the bladder muscles. This often results in stress urinary incontinence—the loss of urine with laughing, coughing, or sneezing. Urinary urgency includes feeling a constant need to urinate. This too is often related to a decrease in estrogen. Just like the vagina, the bladder is an estrogen-sensitive organ, and when estrogen levels drop, bladder symptoms often develop.

Insomnia is the inability to fall asleep or stay asleep for a long enough time to feel rested and rejuvenated. Night sweats, incontinence, and even menopause-related bizarre dreams can contribute to the insomnia.

Anxiety, panic attacks, worry, fear, edginess, unease, and a disproportional sense of urgency are all related to a menopausal drop in hormones, which affects brain chemistry.

Here is a comprehensive list of common symptoms of perimenopause or menopause:

- hot flashes
- night sweats
- vaginal dryness
- anxiety
- panic attacks
- mood swings
- irritability
- insomnia
- weird dreams
- snoring
- depression
- loss of sexual interest
- painful intercourse
- hair loss
- hair growth on face
- urinary tract infections
- aching ankles, knees, wrists, shoulders, heels
- lower back pain
- bloating
- flatulence
- urinary leakage
- indigestion
- osteoporosis
- vaginal itching
- frequent urination
- sore breasts
- palpitations
- varicose veins
- dizzy spells
- skin feeling "crawly"
- migraine headaches
- memory lapses
- weight gain

TESTING, TREATMENT FOR PROGESTERONE

If you are still early enough in the perimenopausal phase of your life that you are having periods, then the optimal time to test your hormone levels is nineteen to twenty-one days after the first day of your period. Often, blood testing will be adequate, though saliva or urine hormone testing is sometimes indicated.

If low progesterone is confirmed, replacement therapy is really the only option for raising the hormone level back to normal, thereby relieving the symptoms you are experiencing. Since the change in hormones is often a fluctuating, unsteady, unpredictable decline during perimenopause, it can be a challenge to get the dosage right when replacing hormones. That's why you need to work with someone who knows what he or she is doing.

Just as with any hormone or medication, side effects can occur when the dosage is too high. With progesterone, the side effects of too much of the hormone in your system are often the same symptoms as too little.

I have had patients come to me on traditional hormone replacement, using Prometrium, a micronized oral progesterone, who showed symptoms of too much progesterone and whose progesterone levels tested very high. Since Prometrium only comes in one dose, allowing for no flexibility if the dosage prescribed is ultimately too high, the problem was resolved by switching to a compounded, slow-release progesterone. The lower dosage brought their progesterone levels down to a more acceptable range and settled their symptoms, confirming that the high progesterone levels were the cause of the problem.

Natural progesterone can be administered in the form of a cream applied to the skin or put into a capsule to take orally.

If you are having trouble sleeping, then progesterone in capsule form is best for you. Taken by mouth, progesterone has all the benefits of the cream form, but it also crosses the blood-brain barrier and directly affects the production of gamma-aminobutyric acid (GABA). Again, the blood-brain barrier blocks some substances from entering your brain while allowing in essential nutrients. GABA is a neurotransmitter that inhibits nerve transmission in the brain, which can calm your nerves, positively impact your mood, and help you achieve better quality and quantity of sleep. If you are falling asleep and then waking at two or three in the morning, unable to go back to sleep, progesterone is your fix.

Progesterone can also be applied in a cream that is rubbed onto your skin once or twice a day. The dosing amount and the number of days you apply the cream is all part of your individualized treatment program.

Typically, improvement from treatment is noticed within the first four weeks. Some women, depending on their symptoms, notice improvement within a week, while others take up to two months to experience any change.

As with any HRT, it is important to arrange a follow-up visit to review your improvement and to perform additional testing to measure your hormone levels.

After you start taking natural progesterone, your own body's production of progesterone will likely continue to decrease. This decline is inevitable and occurs whether or not you use replacement therapy. It's important to understand the implications of this decline: Even if you started on HRT and your symptoms were resolved, they may return, indicating that your dose needs to be increased or that other hormones have started to change. It is important to evaluate your full hormone profile with each follow-up visit to check for optimal values, as well as for changes in other hormone levels.

JEAN

A More Efficient Approach to Better Health

Jean's menopausal symptoms made it difficult to get through a business day without feeling a bit embarrassed. "I spend many hours a day in meetings with clients, our staff, and others, and hot flashes would come without notice," she said. Add to that night sweats that kept her from sleeping and ultimately made her tired and irritable at home and at work. Plus, she had put on weight despite eating a balanced diet and working with a trainer twice a week for years—a factor that led to depression.

With her quality of life drastically reduced, she sought help from George Arnold, MD, at the recommendation of her general practitioner. Dr. Arnold prescribed the combination of progesterone and estrogen, and in a few weeks, Jean's night sweats and hot flashes stopped completely. Soon, she was able to drop the weight she had gained, happily returning to a size two.

"I can honestly say that Dr. Arnold gave me my life back," Jean said. "Dr. Arnold is very pleasant and easy to talk to, and his team is friendly and efficient." Jean added that she appreciated having the bloodwork forms mailed in advance of her appointment, allowing Dr. Arnold to have the results in hand. "It's a shortcut to feeling better, something a person like me, with a very busy schedule, can appreciate," Jean said.

DISPELLING THE MYTHS OF PROGESTERONE

Here are some of the misconceptions that patients bring to me about progesterone and bioidentical hormone replacement.

Q: "Is it possible to overdose on progesterone?"

A: While it's possible to have too little progesterone, an overdose of progesterone is rare. Some people, however, experience mild side effects from too high a dose, including headaches, dizziness, breast pain, urinary problems, nausea, or abdominal pain.[34]

Q: "Will my body stop making progesterone once I start treatment?"

A: Again, taking progesterone will not increase the speed at which your body decreases its own production of progesterone. What you take adds to what your body produces. Your body cannot tell the difference between the progesterone your body produces and the natural progesterone that you take. Both will bind to your progesterone receptors and have the same effect.

PROGESTERONE FOR MEN

Progesterone is also an important hormone in men. Progesterone helps balance estrogen, which can rise to unhealthy levels in aging men. In balancing estrogen in men, progesterone antagonizes the stimulatory effects of estrogen on the

prostate gland. It lowers prostate-specific antigen (PSA), a protein produced by prostate gland cells, and stimulates anti-tumor antigen, which helps prevent prostate cancer.

---

34   Max Whitmore, "Side Effects When You Take Too Much Progesterone," *Livestrong.com* (August 16, 2013), accessed October 16, 2016, http://www.livestrong.com/article/445186-side-effects-when-you-take-too-much-progesterone/.

Progesterone starts to decline in men at around age sixty. Low progesterone symptoms in men include:

- hair loss

- weight gain

- fatigue

- low libido

- depression

- erectile dysfunction, impotence

- gynecomastia, or "man boobs"

- bone, muscle loss

Men with low progesterone levels may also develop arthritis, osteoporosis, and even prostate cancer.

THE DIFFERENCE IS NIGHT AND DAY

"I haven't felt this good in five years. This is like night and day." Those were Jane's comments in her first follow-up visit eight weeks after she began treatment.

Jane's situation was fairly common, starting with progesterone replacement and then, over time, needing to add in estrogen and testosterone. Some women start treatment with all three—progesterone, estrogen, testosterone—and then add in thyroid as well.

Every woman is different, which is why treatment involves an individualized approach. A good oral history, an examination where appropriate, and a full hormone profile from bloodwork, saliva, or urine can help identify which hormones are likely deficient and contributing to the symptoms being experienced.

By listening to Jane and conducting tests, we were able to diagnose her and provide a customized treatment plan.

In the next chapter, I'll discuss HRT for women who are still in their childbearing years. If you're beyond childbearing years, you may find this to be a helpful chapter to share with a daughter, niece, neighbor, or friend.

Chapter 4 Symptom Chart: **Progesterone**

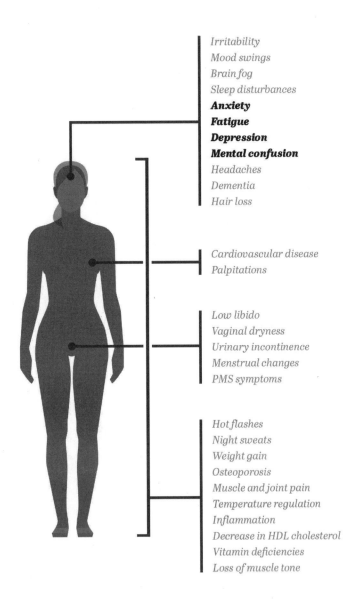

Irritability
Mood swings
Brain fog
Sleep disturbances
Anxiety
Fatigue
Depression
Mental confusion
Headaches
Dementia
Hair loss

Cardiovascular disease
Palpitations

Low libido
Vaginal dryness
Urinary incontinence
Menstrual changes
PMS symptoms

Hot flashes
Night sweats
Weight gain
Osteoporosis
Muscle and joint pain
Temperature regulation
Inflammation
Decrease in HDL cholesterol
Vitamin deficiencies
Loss of muscle tone

Chapter 4

PROGESTERONE: DURING AND POST-PREGNANCY

At age thirty-four, Louise became pregnant with her second child. She had experienced mild postpartum depression following her first delivery three years prior but had taken no medication for the condition at that time. However, during her thirty-week visit to my office, she began complaining of worsening depression. So, I started her on a bioidentical progesterone cream, which she applied to her skin twice a day. Within two weeks of starting the progesterone treatment, her depression had almost entirely cleared.

At her six-week postpartum visit, she remained on the progesterone and was feeling fine. She had no postpartum depression at all. She continued for two more months and then tapered off the medication.

PROGESTERONE PRODUCTION FOR PREGNANCY

Progesterone plays a crucial role in fetal development during pregnancy.

In the previous chapter, I mentioned how progesterone prepares the uterus for pregnancy by thickening the uterine lining to create a supportive environment in which to implant and grow the fertilized egg. Once the egg is fertilized, progesterone continues to provide a nurturing environment. At approximately eight to ten weeks, the ovaries pass production of progesterone on to the placenta. At this point, progesterone substantially increases to help strengthen the wall muscles of the pelvis in preparation for the labor to come.

In a regulating role, progesterone also stimulates breast tissue during pregnancy while preventing lactation. During and immediately following pregnancy, the hormone prolactin is secreted by the pituitary gland to stimulate breast development and milk production. Breastfeeding following birth then significantly lowers progesterone levels until the mother stops lactating, at which point prolactin levels decline and progesterone levels begin to rise again.

Often, if a woman can conceive but has trouble carrying to term, it's because of progesterone production. If there's not enough progesterone being produced during the first two to three months of the pregnancy, it can impact the ability of the pregnancy to continue. During that time frame, the main progesterone production comes from the ovaries. Miscarriages or interruptions in development sometimes occur between six and eight weeks, often because there isn't enough progesterone to keep the pregnancy going until the placenta takes over production of progesterone at around the ten-week mark.

Hormone replacement treatment for women having problems conceiving and for those with recurrent miscarriages is intended to provide progesterone support until the pregnancy successfully reaches twelve weeks.

Progesterone has been used extensively and safely in the first trimester and throughout pregnancy.

DEALING WITH POSTPARTUM DEPRESSION

Postpartum depression (PPD), also known as postnatal depression (PND), is defined as "the first occurrence of psychiatric symptoms severe enough to require medical help occurring after childbirth and before the return of menstruation."[35]

When a woman conceives, carries a fetus, gives birth, breast-feeds, and then returns to a post-pregnancy condition, her hormones undergo significant change. While not all women will have trouble with hormonal imbalance following pregnancy, those who do should seek help as soon as possible. With HRT, returning to a happy, healthy post-pregnancy state is possible.

In her groundbreaking 2001 book *Depression after Childbirth: How to Recognise, Treat, and Prevent Postnatal Depression*, British physician Katharina Dalton reported the following rate of incidences in new mothers following childbirth:

- **Eight in ten women feel "the baby blues."** This feeling of sadness, moodiness, and weepiness is short-lived, typically lasting only a few weeks. Other symptoms of "the baby blues" may include fatigue, poor concentration, confusion, and mild anxiety. Sometimes, an expectant mother will develop asthma or headaches during pregnancy that disappear in the third trimester. However, these symptoms may return in full force in the first week following childbirth. [36]

- **One in ten experience postpartum depression.** When the tears continue to flow after a few weeks, it's likely that "the baby blues" are actually something more long term

35   Katharina Dalton with Wendy Holton, *Depression after Childbirth: How to Recognise, Treat, and Prevent Postnatal Illness* (Oxford: Oxford University Press, 2001).

36   Ibid.

and potentially more serious—but still treatable. Half of women receiving treatment were still depressed one year after giving birth. Thirty percent of women who received no treatment were still depressed three years after giving birth.[37]

- **One in two hundred experience puerperal psychosis.** For some women, the depression following childbirth is extremely serious. Psychotic symptoms may come on suddenly and include extreme irritability, wild mood swings, or even hallucinations. Other early signs of psychosis may include personality changes, delusions, a disconnect with reality, or suicidal thoughts or comments. Some new mothers require psychiatric hospitalization for their symptoms. The onset of psychosis often occurs immediately after labor or overnight. Early warning signs of psychosis are anxiety and insomnia.[38]

- **One in 125,000 will commit infanticide.** When a solution such as HRT exists, PPD should never reach this level of severity.

Early symptoms of PPD may include selective hearing, anxiety, constant crying, general feelings of sadness, agitation or irritability, trouble concentrating, confusion, feeling worthless, or losing interest in activities that you commonly do every day. Some women also experience guilt or a lack of interest or outright rejection of their new baby. And some find themselves completely frustrated over feelings

---

37   David McNamee, "How long does postpartum depression last?" *Medical News Today.com* (July 13, 2015), accessed October 16, 2016, http://www.medicalnewstoday.com/articles/271217.php.

38   Katharina Dalton with Wendy Holton, *Depression after Childbirth: How to Recognise, Treat, and Prevent Postnatal Illness* (Oxford: Oxford University Press, 2001).

of incompetence or inadequacy when it comes to coping with or caring for their baby.

Changes in sleeping or eating habits can be early signs of PPD. Insomnia or oversleeping and yet feeling extremely fatigued—physically and mentally—can be signs of PPD.

A change in eating habits can also signal a problem. Often, a woman's appetite will increase, and she'll have odd cravings. She will eat high-calorie foods, and within a few months of giving birth, she'll be heavier than her top pregnancy weight.

PPD women usually feel best upon waking, but as the day wears on, their condition worsens. They become irritable and more depressed. They are exhausted and, after eating a high-calorie snack, just want to go to bed.[39]

IT'S A MEDICAL—NOT MENTAL—ISSUE

The key with postpartum depression is to remember that *it is not a psychological condition*. Postpartum depression is *caused by a hormonal imbalance*. That message bears repeating: Hormonal imbalance following pregnancy is behind the depression, mood swings, and psychological disturbances many women feel after giving birth.

Exhaustion, a PPD-like symptom, can also be caused by medical issues such as low thyroid (again, a hormonal imbalance), anemia, and low potassium.[40]

Unfortunately, new mothers often wait weeks to get an appointment with a psychiatrist because postpartum depression is not typically viewed as an urgent matter. But that is exactly the problem. While it is usually a temporary condition, its effects can be very

39 Ibid.
40 Ibid.

intense, so postpartum depression should be treated with a sense of urgency.

In addition to being linked to PPD symptoms, a drop in progesterone is also linked to premenstrual syndrome (PMS), that time prior to menstruation when many women experience symptoms ranging from water retention and physical aches and pains to irritability and mood swings. With the drop in progesterone comes a rise in estrogen, which can lead to PMS symptoms. Progesterone replacement to correct hormonal imbalance can help treat PMS symptoms, relieving the tiredness and tension that, for some women, is a monthly occurrence.

Progesterone replacement is a far better solution for PMS than a hysterectomy, since menstrual hormones are not controlled by the ovaries but by the menstrual-system control region of the hypothalamus.

As I've discussed in previous chapters, the hypothalamus is an important regulator, located in the lower part of the brain. Among the body components that the hypothalamus controls are your menstrual system and the pregnancy hormones FSH (follicle-stimulating hormone) and LH (luteinizing hormone). Where FSH stimulates the egg to grow in the ovary, LH causes the egg to release, making it available for fertilization. The hypothalamus also controls the hormones estrogen and progesterone and—as part of the menstrual system—mood, body weight, and wake/sleep rhythm. Progesterone receptors, meanwhile, are largely concentrated in the emotional center of the brain known as the limbic area. However, as I've mentioned, other receptor sites are also located throughout your body—in your eyes, nasal passages, lungs, liver, bones, and urethra; and in your breasts, vagina, and uterus, as well. When childbirth causes abrupt declines in the hypothalamic hormones, you can probably see why you experience disruptions in your moods, weight, and wake/sleep cycles, which can result in PPD.

Progesterone also aids in inhibiting the buildup of monoamine oxidase, an enzyme that removes the mood-enhancing neurotransmitters serotonin, dopamine, and norepinephrine from the brain. While serotonin manages appetite, mood, and sleep, dopamine is known as a reward and pleasure stimulant, and norepinephrine is a motivator that aids focus and alertness.

DENA

Getting Off the Roller Coaster

After having her second child at age thirty-seven, Dena decided not to go back on birth control. By that time, she'd been on birth control for more than twenty years, and since her husband underwent a vasectomy, she decided she might be better off without.

Before long, however, Dena found herself dealing with a roller coaster of symptoms. She had intense, debilitating migraines prior to menstruation, and her periods became erratically spaced with inconsistent flow. Her moods became uncontrollable, which was atypical for her. "I was completely stressed out," Dena said. "I quit my job and decided to be a stay-at-home mom. Still, I was no longer the happy person I had been."

Worst of all, Dena said, her sleep became disrupted to the point of ending altogether. "At first, I could not fall asleep. Then I could not stay asleep. All my life, I was an eight-hours-a-night sleeper. But I started sleeping only three or four hours a night."

Dena's family physician put her back on birth control, which relieved some of her symptoms. But what her doctor identified as premenstrual syndrome, Dena was convinced was something else. "I thought it had to be declining hormones, even though my doctor did bloodwork and insisted I wasn't going through perimenopause," she said.

Dena struggled with her symptoms for several years. During that time, she researched bioidentical hormones but was afraid to switch from birth control even though her prescription wasn't relieving her symptoms. When her doctor's practice moved, Dena began shopping around and came across Signature Hormones online. "Finally, I had some hope," she said.

When Dr. Arnold ordered different bloodwork than her family physician had ordered, Dena felt certain she was on the right track. Her lab results along with her initial consultation confirmed that she was indeed in perimenopause. Within days of beginning treatment of estrogen, progesterone, DHEA, and testosterone, Dena began feeling better. "The progesterone was a lifesaver for me as I could then sleep through the night! After seven years of insomnia, it was good to be able to sleep again." Dena's migraines, other aches and pains, and emotional roller coaster all came to an end. "I feel like a million bucks!" she said. "Dr. Arnold is kind, helpful, and generous with his time. Most importantly, he knows about female issues and knows how to get a woman on the path to feeling well. I couldn't recommend a more perfect doctor to help women with these delicate issues later in life."

TREATMENT WITH PROGESTERONE
DURING PREGNANCY

To date, no data from randomized controlled trials (RCTs) and other studies for prevention of preterm birth indicate progesterone therapy as unsafe. Progesterone may be prescribed on the basis that it has been found to help with symptoms, and there are no risks to either the fetus or the mother from using it.

In fact, studies have found that progesterone administered during pregnancy can actually reduce other health risks.

A 2002 study measuring third-trimester progesterone levels and the maternal risk of breast cancer found that increasing levels of progesterone were associated with a decreased risk of breast cancer.[41] Subjects in the study with the highest progesterone levels had a 50 percent reduction in the incidence of breast cancer, and the association was stronger for cancers diagnosed at or before age fifty.

A 1999 study also found that women who experience preeclampsia—a risky condition marked by high blood pressure and high levels of protein in the urine, typically occurring after the twenty-week mark in a pregnancy—may actually have a reduced risk for breast cancer.[42] That's because preeclampsia is associated with an elevation in progesterone levels.

In the last few years, the use of natural hormones has expanded to include treatment for infertility, to prevent miscarriages, to reduce the risk of threatened preterm labor, and to treat women found to have a shortened cervix after twenty weeks of gestation, which can lead to preterm labor.

---

41   Jennifer David Peck, et al., "Steroid Hormone Levels During Pregnancy and Incidence of Maternal Breast Cancer," *Cancer Epidemiology, Biomarkers & Prevention* 11, no. 4 (April 2002): 361-8, accessed October 16, 2016, http://cebp.aacrjournals.org/content/11/4/361.long.

42   K. E. Innes and T. E. Byers, "Preeclampsia and breast cancer risk," *Epidemiology* 10, no. 6 (November 1999): 722-32, accessed on U.S. National Library of Medicine National Institutes of Health, October 16, 2016, https://www.ncbi.nlm.nih.gov/pubmed/10535787.

Before administering progesterone, diet and other factors must be addressed, since progesterone does not bind to its receptors when sugar levels are low or adrenaline levels are high.

"Normal" progesterone ranges fluctuate, so measuring your progesterone level during pregnancy does not help in diagnosing low progesterone. However, at the end of a pregnancy, it's common to see progesterone levels drop from around 150 ng/ml (nanograms per milliliter) to less than 7 ng/ml within days of giving birth, to being immeasurable within a week after childbirth.[43]

Since blood levels in the first eight to twelve weeks aren't the best indicators of normal progesterone levels, diagnosis also involves observation.

One effective tool for diagnosing PPD is the Edinburgh Postnatal Depression Scale (EPDS). The EPDS is a ten-question, self-rating test for women who are pregnant or have recently given birth to a child to determine whether they are at risk for PPD. The test looks at how a woman felt in the seven days prior to taking the test and asks the taker to respond with one of four choices that gauge the occurrence of the act in question, from "most of the time" to "never."

A few sample questions on the EPDS include:[44]

- "I have been able to laugh and see the funny side of things."

- "I have looked forward with enjoyment to things."

- "I have blamed myself unnecessarily when things went wrong."

- "I have been anxious or worried for no good reason."

---

43   Katharina Dalton with Wendy Holton, *Depression after Childbirth: How to Recognise, Treat, and Prevent Postnatal Illness* (Oxford: Oxford University Press, 2001).

44   "Edinburgh Postnatal Depression Scale (EPDS)," American Academy of Pediatrics, accessed October 16, 2016, http://www2.aap.org/sections/scan/practicingsafety/toolkit_resources/module2/epds.pdf.

Since PPD and PMS are associated with a drop in progesterone, replacement therapy is also effective as a preventive treatment for recurrence of PPD in women who experience severe PMS. As a preventive treatment, progesterone can also help women who have a history of PPD and whose immediate family member (mother, sister, aunt) experienced PPD. For these women, progesterone may be administered immediately after giving birth, before the onset of PPD symptoms, as a way of averting the effects resulting from the abrupt drop in progesterone that typically occurs upon delivery. Administering replacement progesterone early on can help hormones gradually return to normal levels until menstruation begins again.[45]

Administering progesterone during pregnancy for treatment of pregnancy-onset depression is also effective and safe.

DISPELLING THE MYTHS OF PROGESTERONE

Here are some of the misconceptions that patients bring to me about progesterone and bioidentical replacement in pregnancy.

Q: "I heard these aren't safe when I'm breastfeeding."
A: There are no concerns about progesterone treatments and breastfeeding.

Q: If I take progesterone, I can't take any other medication, can I?
A: Progesterone does not interact with any other medication.

STILL PRODUCING

Having succeeded on HRT with her second pregnancy, Louise came to me when she was pregnant with her third child. The third time

---

45   Katharina Dalton with Wendy Holton, *Depression after Childbirth: How to Recognise, Treat, and Prevent Postnatal Illness* (Oxford: Oxford University Press, 2001).

around, her depression started around week twenty-five, as opposed to week thirty. As soon as her depression started, we performed the necessary tests and then added the progesterone cream in the same dosage as we had with her second pregnancy, and it worked just as well as it had the previous time.

The best way to resolve PPD is to treat the cause, not just the symptoms. With traditional medicine, the most common treatment for postpartum depression is antidepressants, which address only the symptom and not the cause. Treatment with progesterone typically involves a cream rubbed on the skin. This simple treatment can make a big difference in emotional swings and can begin to address the cause of PPD, typically within a week.

Progesterone dosages potentially need to be one thousand times greater than any accompanying estrogen. So, now let's talk about that vital hormone in your body—estrogen.

Chapter 5 Symptom Chart: **Estrogen**

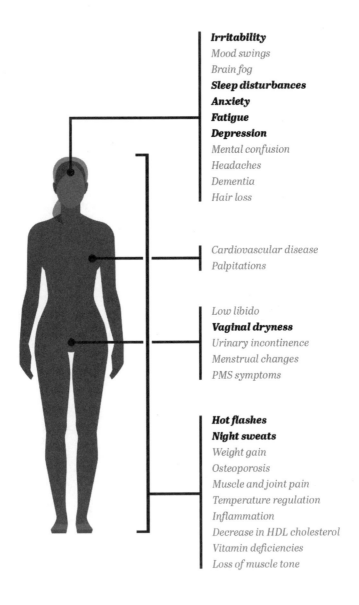

Irritability
Mood swings
Brain fog
Sleep disturbances
Anxiety
Fatigue
Depression
Mental confusion
Headaches
Dementia
Hair loss

Cardiovascular disease
Palpitations

Low libido
Vaginal dryness
Urinary incontinence
Menstrual changes
PMS symptoms

Hot flashes
Night sweats
Weight gain
Osteoporosis
Muscle and joint pain
Temperature regulation
Inflammation
Decrease in HDL cholesterol
Vitamin deficiencies
Loss of muscle tone

Chapter 5

ESTROGEN: FOR THE BEST YOU

At age fifty-seven, Lisa had been experiencing symptoms of menopause—hot flashes, night sweats, trouble sleeping, and decreased libido.

Her lab tests revealed she was experiencing menopause. She had elevated follicle-stimulating hormone (FSH) levels and low levels of estradiol, progesterone, and free testosterone. I initially started her on a cream made of Bi-Est and progesterone. Bi-Est is composed of two estrogens: estriol, a weak form of estrogen, and estradiol, a strong form of estrogen.

Eight weeks after she started treatment, she came in for a follow-up visit. Her hot flashes and night sweats had completely disappeared and she was sleeping beautifully.

THE FUNCTION OF ESTROGENS

Now we come to what most people think of first when talking about women's hormones—estrogen. As a member of "The Best-Me Club," you've no doubt been dealing with changing levels of the estrogens in your body.

To recap, estrogens are hormones produced naturally in your body that are key to sexual development and other functions of your body.

When you're still experiencing a menstrual cycle, estrogen is made primarily in your ovaries by the eggs that develop there each month. Estrogen production falls off when your ovaries stop producing eggs, which occurs naturally with age or because of surgical removal of the ovaries. As soon as a woman's supply of eggs has ended, estrogen levels start to go down. Once you enter menopause, most estrogen in your body is made in your adrenal gland and in your fat cells.

Like your other hormones, the estrogens in your body are mostly bound to either sex-hormone-binding globulin (SHBG) or albumin, two hormones made primarily by the liver. Only about 1 percent of your estrogen is free or unbound. The unbound estrogen works in your body by crossing into your cells and binding to estrogen receptors. Women have estrogen receptors in just about every organ and tissue: the brain, eyes, heart, gut, breasts, muscles, bone, bladder, intestines, uterus, vagina, lungs, and blood vessels. To obtain the ultimate biologic response when taking HRT, you must use hormones that your body has receptors for. That's where bioidentical hormones come in.

Think about it: Premarin is one of the most common estrogen medications in use for the last few decades. Yet, Premarin is made up of horse estrogen, known as equilin. How many receptors in your body do you think are designed to bind with horse estrogen? None. Put another way: If you were to need a blood transfusion, how well do you think horse blood would work?

ESTROGEN IS GOOD FOR YOU

Since women have estrogen receptors throughout their bodies, it's no wonder estrogen plays such a vital role in a woman's health.

For instance, estrogen aids in cardiovascular health, reducing the risk of heart disease by up to 50 percent. It does so by helping to maintain the elasticity of arteries and dilating small arteries. It also keeps platelets in the blood from sticking and decreases plaque accumulation on arteries. Estrogen raises good cholesterol (HDL) by up to 15 percent and lowers lipoproteins, which are soluble proteins that transport fat molecules in the blood. Estrogen also acts as a natural calcium channel blocker to keep arteries open.

In the brain, estrogen boosts N-methyl-D-aspartate receptors (NMDA)—boosting long-term memory—by 30 percent. Estrogen decreases the risk of Alzheimer's by up to 40 percent. The longer you are on estrogen, the lower your risk of developing Alzheimer's. Estrogen enhances dopamine's ability to aid in motor function, and it increases the availability of acetylcholine, the neurotransmitter of memory. Since estrogen has a direct influence on the amount of serotonin produced—remember, serotonin is the feel-good hormone responsible for appetite, mood, and sleep—declining estrogen levels in menopause resulting in lower serotonin production can lead to mood swings, sadness and depression, foggy thinking, fluctuation of appetite, loss of sleep, and even thoughts of suicide. Estrogen increases the levels of gamma-aminobutyric acid (GABA) in your system. From earlier in the book, you know that GABA can calm your nerves and positively impact your mood, and it plays an important role in both sleep quality and quantity.

One of the most noticeable changes in estrogen levels manifests in skin tone and appearance. Estrogen helps maintain collagen and increases the water content of skin. Looking at women in their fifties, sixties, seventies, I can typically tell who is taking hormones and who is not. Those who are tend to have glowing skin. They have fewer wrinkles. They have better skin tone.

In fact, estrogen has over four hundred different functions in the body, including:

- regulates body temperature

- improves metabolic rate

- enhances sleep

- improves muscle tone, lessens muscle damage

- stimulates enzymes that prevent Alzheimer's disease

- improves insulin sensitivity

- helps with magnesium absorption

- boosts energy, mood, and concentration

- maintains bone density

- increases sexual interest

- protects against cataracts and macular degeneration

- decreases risk of colon cancer

- helps prevent tooth loss

KARIN

Relief for Menopause

Karin was in her fifties when she began to suffer from symptoms of menopause: frequent night sweats, mood changes, and sleeplessness. "I was miserable," Karin said. "The night sweats soaked my nightclothes, my hair, my sheets.

And the lack of sleep affected my days. Plus, although they weren't as intense as the night sweats, I was starting to have hot flashes during the day."

A cousin referred Karin to Dr. Arnold, and after she did her own research on Signature Hormones and bioidentical HRT, she decided to make an appointment to see him. "He talked with me about my symptoms, and then after he got the lab results from my bloodwork, he prescribed bioidentical estrogen, progesterone, and testosterone in cream form," she said. "It took a few weeks for my symptoms to begin to subside, but as my hormones started to get back to normal levels, I began to experience relief fairly quickly."

As a result, Karin reported, she began to sleep well, and her other symptoms had completely gone.

"What I appreciated most about Dr. Arnold's care was that he took the time to ask me questions and then carefully review my lab results before putting together a prescription based on my personal hormone levels," Karin said. "I appreciate how efficiently he worked, and how he was both professional and personable in the way he related to me. Anyone seeing Dr. Arnold for help would find themselves in excellent hands. I wish I had known him during my childbearing years!"

THREE ESTROGENS AT WORK

Did you know that your body produces not one, but three estrogens? That's right, they are: estrone (E1), estradiol (E2), and estriol (E3). Prior to menopause, estradiol is the predominant estrogen your body

ces; after menopause, it's estrone. Let's look at the three and
effect they have on your body.

Estrone (E1)

Before you enter menopause, estrone is made by your ovaries, adrenal glands, liver, and fat cells. In your ovaries, estrone converts to estradiol until you're postmenopausal, at which time very little conversion takes place. In postmenopause, the main source of estrone is fat. Therefore, the more fat your body has, the more estrone you make. Research has shown that high levels of estrone may increase a woman's risk of both breast cancer and endometrial (uterine lining) cancer.

Estradiol (E2)

Estradiol is the strongest form of estrogen. It helps protect your heart, bones, brain, and nervous system. It is the main hormone produced by your body prior to menopause. Like estrone, estradiol is also produced primarily in your ovaries. Even postmenopause, two-thirds of women who still have their ovaries will continue to make small amounts of estradiol. In fact, most women continue to make some estradiol into their eighties.

In women, estradiol is beneficial in increasing levels of good cholesterol (HDL) while lowering bad cholesterol (LDL) and total cholesterol. Estradiol also lowers triglycerides, the most common form of body fat and the main ingredient in animal fats and vegetable oils. Although triglycerides provide your cells with metabolic energy, high levels of triglycerides can lead to coronary heart disease, diabetes, and fatty liver.[46]

---

46 "Triglycerides: Frequently Asked Questions," American Heart Association/American Stroke Association, accessed November 12, 2016, http://www.heart.org/idc/groups/ahamah-public/(@wcm/(@sop/(@smd/documents/downloadable/ucm_425988.pdf.

Estradiol helps maintain bone structure through a remodeling process, employing an action known as "resorption." The bones in your body are not static. They are made of living tissue, which is constantly being broken down and rebuilt.[47] The cells that break down old bone tissue are known as osteoclasts, and the cells that build new bone tissue are known as osteoblasts. There's a balance to the process that is affected by estrogen levels.

Osteoporosis, sometimes known as brittle-bone disease, is a change in bone-mineral density, often because of a change in estrogen levels. Studies have found a link between imbalanced estrogen levels and osteoporosis, citing higher formation of osteoclasts and higher rates of resorption.

Estrogen doesn't have any effect on osteoblasts. It doesn't help build bone. That's the role of progesterone. However, estradiol does help slow the bone-dissolving activity of osteoclasts by inhibiting a substance known as cytokines. Cytokines are protein molecules released by cells that aid in cell communication and stimulate cells to respond to sites of inflammation, trauma, and infection in your body. One cytokine in particular, interleukin-6 (IL-6), activates osteoclasts.[48] When estradiol levels are low, IL-6 levels rise. Estrogen replacement can keep IL-6 at bay and return balance to the bone-remodeling process in your body.

In the brain, estradiol increases the production of some neurotransmitters, including serotonin, the body's appetite, mood, and sleep enhancer; acetylcholine, which is associated with memory; dopamine, which is associated with movement, motivation, and

---

47   Xu Feng and Jay McDonald, "Disorders of Bone Remodeling," *Annual Review of Pathology Mechanisms of Disease* 6 (2011): 121-145, accessed on National Library of Medicine National Institutes of Health, November 10, 2016, https://www.ncbi.nlm.nih.gov/pmc/articles/PMC3571087/.

48   Ibid.

reward; and norepinephrine, or noradrenaline, which increases mental alertness.

Low estradiol can lead to sleep disturbances that can manifest in daytime fatigue. Estradiol also works as an antioxidant to reduce inflammation, and it helps absorption of calcium, magnesium, and zinc.

Estriol (E3)

Estriol is the least potent estrogen. It is eighty times weaker than estradiol and does not offer the heart, bone, or brain protection that estradiol does. However, estriol is considered safer than both estrone and estradiol. It has even been shown to protect against breast cancer and to decrease the reoccurrence of breast cancer.

Among the studies demonstrating estriol's protective nature against cancer are:

- Lyytinen (2006): No risk of breast cancer was detected in women given oral estriol for at least six months from 1994 to 2001.[49]

- Siiteri (2002): A study of fifteen thousand women found that those who had high levels of estriol during pregnancy had a 58 percent lower breast-cancer risk forty years later.[50]

- Takahashi (2000): A study of fifty-three postmenopausal women who were given 2 mg of oral estriol per day for twelve months found no indications of cancer in either

---

49 H. Lyytinen, E. Pukkala, and O. Ylikorkala, "Breast cancer risk in postmenopausal women using estrogen-only therapy," *Obstetrics and Gynecology* 108, no. 6 (December 2006): 1354-60, accessed on National Library of Medicine National Institutes of Health, November 20, 2016, https://www.ncbi.nlm.nih.gov/pubmed/17138766.

50 Siiteri, P., et. al., "Prospective study of estrogens during pregnancy and risk of breast cancer," Public Health Institute, findings presented at Department of Defense Breast Cancer Research Meeting, September 26, 2002, http://www.lifeextension.com/magazine/2008/8/estriol-its-weakness-is-its-strength/page-01?p=1.

endometrial or breast tissue. The women had gone through either natural or surgically induced menopause.[51]

Estriol can help control symptoms of menopause. It lowers bacteria and restores pH in the vagina.[52] A study in which 0.5 mg of estriol was administered daily for two weeks, and then twice a week for another eight months, found that the dose reduced incidences of urinary tract infections.[53] Another study of eighty-eight women given 2-mg-estriol suppositories at the same frequency found that 68 percent saw improvement in their incontinence symptoms.[54] By maintaining favorable conditions in your gastrointestinal tract, estriol also helps the growth of beneficial gut bacteria, lactobacilli.[55]

Since estriol is produced by the placenta, increasing levels of estriol during pregnancy are an indication that a baby in the womb is developing healthily.

Estriol binds to estrogen receptors and, once there, blocks its stronger sister, estradiol, from doing its work. Estriol has some anti-cancerous properties, particularly when it blocks breast-cancer-cell receptor sites. Synthetic estrogens that are administered as part of HRT are typically composed of high doses of estrone or estradiol

51   K. Takahashi, et al., "Safety and efficacy of oestriol for symptoms of natural or surgically induced menopause," *Human Reproduction* 15, no. 5 (May 2000): 1028-36, abstract accessed on National Library of Medicine National Institutes of Health, November 20, 2016, https://www.ncbi.nlm.nih.gov/pubmed/10783346.

52   Cihat Ünlü and Gilbert Donders, "Use of lactobacilli and estriol combination in the treatment of disturbed vaginal ecosystem: a review," *Journal of the Turkish German Gynecological Association* 12, no. 4 (2011): 239-246, accessed on National Library of Medicine National Institutes of Health, November 20, 2016, https://www.ncbi.nlm.nih.gov/pmc/articles/PMC3939257/, doi: 10.5152/jtgga.2011.57.

53   R. Raz and W. E. Stamm, "A controlled trial of intravaginal estriol in postmenopausal women with recurrent urinary tract infections," *The New England Journal of Medicine* 329, no. 11 (September 9, 1993): 753-6, abstract accessed on National Library of Medicine National Institutes of Health, November 20, 2016, https://www.ncbi.nlm.nih.gov/pubmed/8350884.

54   S. Dessole, et al., "Efficacy of low-dose intravaginal estriol on urogenital aging in postmenopausal women," *Menopause* 11, no. 1 (January 2004): 49-56, abstract accessed on National Library of Medicine National Institutes of Health, November 20, 2016, https://www.ncbi.nlm.nih.gov/pubmed/14716182.

55   "Lactobacillus," U.S. National Library of Medicine, *MedlinePlus.gov*, accessed November 20, 2016, https://medlineplus.gov/druginfo/natural/790.html.

along with little or no estriol. That combination can throw off the natural balance of estrogen in your body.

HOW ESTROGEN IS BROKEN DOWN BY YOUR BODY

Before and during menopause, estradiol (E2) converts to estrone (E1) through a process involving progesterone and the enzyme 17 beta-hydroxysteroid dehydrogenase (HSD). Enzymes are molecules, typically composed of proteins, that occur naturally in your body.

Estrone then converts into the three metabolites: 2-hydroxyestrone, 16-alpha-hydroxyestrone, and 4-hydroxyestrone. "Hydroxy" simply describes the elemental makeup of the metabolite: two parts hydrogen for each one part oxygen—the same makeup as water molecules.

Metabolites are, in essence, molecules that are formed by reactions within your cells. Those cellular reactions are spurred on by enzymes.[56] Each of the three estrogen metabolites can be found in different ratios in your body, and each has its own function.

2-hydroxyestrone

The metabolite 2-hydroxyestrone has very weak estrogenic activity, but is protective against breast cancer. It is also a potent antioxidant that researchers believe can curtail the development and progression of disease. For instance, 2-hydroxyestrone protects against athero-sclerosis, which is a slow hardening and narrowing of the arteries. High levels of 2-hydroxyestrone in your blood are associated with low levels of atherosclerosis.

---

56   Edward D. Harris, "Biochemical Facts behind the Definition and Properties of Metabolites," Texas A&M University, http://www.fda.gov/ohrms/dockets/ac/03/briefing/3942b1_08_Harris%20Paper.pdf.

The 2-hydroxyestrone metabolite can be methylated, or molecularly bound, to 2-methoxyestrone, a metabolite that protects against breast cancer in women (and prostate cancer in men). "Methoxy" is another descriptor of metabolite makeup, which in this case means methane gas bound to oxygen. Studies are now looking at 2-methoxyestrogens for use in treating breast cancer and cardiovascular disease.[57]

At Signature, we can get an idea of how well your estrogen is being methylated to good metabolites by measuring the level of homocysteine—an amino acid—in your blood. Amino acids are protein building blocks and cell metabolizers. When you consume a protein, it is broken down into amino acids that then form new proteins with specific functions such as moving your body's molecules around, aiding in cell communication, and acting as enzymes to speed up the rate of chemical reactions that occur within your cells. Having elevated levels of homocysteine in your bloodstream—a condition known as hyperhomocysteinemia—may indicate the presence of atherosclerosis and blood clots. More commonly though, higher homocysteine levels typically indicate a problem with the way your estrogen is being broken down, or methylated, and can indicate an increased risk for developing breast cancer. At Signature, this condition can be easily treated, thereby reducing your risk.

16-alpha-hydroxyestrone

Strong estrogenic activity is the hallmark of the metabolite 16-alpha-hydroxyestrone. This metabolite turns on estrogen receptors, and high levels of 16-alpha-hydroxyestrone are associated with estrogen-dependent conditions. Estrogen-dependent conditions are disorders

---

57   Raghvendra Dubey, Bruno Imthurn, and Edwin K. Jackson, "2-Methoxyestradiol: A Potential Treatment for Multiple Proliferative Disorders," *Endocrinology* 148, issue 9, (2007), accessed November 21, 2016, http://press.endocrine.org/doi/full/10.1210/en.2007-0514.

that rely on or are sensitive to estrogen levels in your body. Some estrogen-dependent conditions include breast pain or tenderness (also called mastodynia or mastalgia), breast fibromas or uterine fibroids, and breast or uterine cancers and endometriosis.

Estrogen metabolites can be measured in your urine, a test that can be done at Signature. The ratio of 2-hydroxyestrone to 16-alpha-hydroxyestrone is important because a low ratio is associated with an increased risk of breast and prostate cancer and with an increased risk of lupus. A high ratio is associated with an increased risk of bone loss.

4-hydroxyestrone

The metabolite 4-hydroxyestrone is a potent estrogen. High levels of 4-hydroxyestrone are associated with an increased risk of breast and prostate cancer, potentially damaging DNA and causing mutations. Women with fibroids tend to have high levels of 4-hydroxyestrone. Also, conjugated equine estrogens such as Premarin break down into 4-hydroxyestrone—one of the reasons I prefer to prescribe bioidentical estrogen.

ESTROGEN IMBALANCES

As with any hormone, too much estrogen can have a negative impact on your body. When there's an imbalance in your estrogen levels, cells are less able to resist infection, and proper function can decrease.

The world we live in today is estrogen-dominant. It's filled with chemicals that act like the hormone estrogen that's in your body. These chemicals are known as xenoestrogens. Dozens of xenoestrogens in our environment—found in pesticides, plastics, cosmetics, and animal feed—imitate estrogen and can be toxic to your body. For instance, antibiotics used on "food animals" can potentially change your gut flora, which are the microorganisms that live in your digestive tract. Also known as microbiota, healthy gut flora keeps your digestive system in balance and helps your body absorb nutrients, vitamins, and minerals. Such antibiotics can change the way your body absorbs and utilizes estrogen and can ultimately lead to breast cancer.[58] Alcohol can also interfere with your body's ability to metabolize estrogen and can raise estradiol levels.

Low estrogen can cause those symptoms associated with menopause—night sweats, hot flashes, and incontinence. Vaginal dryness is also a symptom of low estrogen. Vaginal dryness may start as itching, irritation, or a burning sensation. Over time, vaginal dryness may cause pain during sex, which can lead to a decrease in libido. When intercourse becomes painful, many women want to avoid it altogether.

Vaginal lubrication can also be affected by low estrogen. Vaginal lubrication problems can occur at any age but seem to be a symptom affecting menopausal and postpartum women the most. Interestingly, the lubrication for sex comes from the vagina, not from the cervix or the uterus. Estrogen thickens vagina walls and produces lubrication. When estrogen levels fall, those functions are affected. In addition to menopause, the ovaries produce less estrogen during the postpartum period and while breastfeeding.

Estrogen has these beneficial effects on your heart: raising good cholesterol while lowering the bad, dilating blood vessels to improve blood flow, and soaking up harmful particles in the blood that damage arteries and tissues.

---

58   S. L. Gorbach, "Estrogens, breast cancer, and intestinal flora," *Reviews of Infectious Diseases* 6, supplement 1 (March-April 1984): S85-90, supplement abstract accessed on U.S. National Library of Medicine National Institutes of Health, November 22, 2016, https://www.ncbi.nlm.nih.gov/pubmed/6326245.

Declining estrogen levels can disrupt your menstruation cycle, leading to what is known as absent menstruation, or amenorrhea. If you miss at least three periods in a row, you have amenorrhea.

Conversely, when estrogen builds up, it can lead to what is known as estrogen dominance, causing health issues ranging from moodiness to breast cysts.

Breast cancer is a concern with elevated estrogen levels. Since roughly two out of three breast-cancer cells have receptors that readily attach to estrogen, high levels of estrogen can promote the spread of breast cancer.[59] Higher breast density has also been found to be an indicator of heightened breast-cancer risk, and studies have found that estrogen may increase breast density.[60]

High estrogen levels have been pointed to as the underlying cause of premenstrual syndrome (PMS), which occurs in the days leading up to the onset of menstruation. Elevated estrogen levels can also lead to menorrhagia, the medical term for menstrual periods with abnormally heavy or prolonged bleeding. Menorrhagia can occur during perimenopause.

High estrogen levels raise your risk of endometrial cancer, or cancer of the uterus, and of endometrial hyperplasia, a precancerous thickening of the uterine lining. High estrogen can also lead to the development of uterine fibroids, benign tumors that grow in the muscle layer of the uterus, and can cause painful periods and other symptoms. Giving medication to decrease the production of estrogen while increasing the amount of progesterone that's available can be quite effective in helping treat fibroids and endometriosis.

---

59   "Hormone Therapy for Breast Cancer," American Cancer Society, accessed November 22, 2016, http://www.cancer.org/cancer/breastcancer/detailedguide/breast-cancer-treating-hormone-therapy.

60   N. F. Boyd, et al., "Mammographic density and the risk and detection of breast cancer," *New England Journal of Medicine* 356, no. 3 (January 18, 2007): 227-36, abstract accessed on National Library of Medicine National Institutes of Health, November 22, 2016, https://www.ncbi.nlm.nih.gov/pubmed/17229950.

When estrogen and progesterone production are imbalanced in your body, you can end up with an excess of estrogen. In severe cases, an imbalance in estrogen and progesterone levels in your body can sometimes lead to surgery—a hysterectomy or ovary removal—which is potentially unnecessary. That's why, when seeking HRT, it is crucial to work with a provider who truly knows how to return balance to your body's hormones.

MARIA

Customized Treatments Reawakened Her Former Self

Maria had suffered through very heavy menstrual cycles since her late thirties but couldn't find answers through a gynecologist. She was also plagued by low blood pressure, blood sugar, and iron levels, and she had difficulty concentrating and was gaining weight. She was tired and irritable, and her low energy levels made it difficult to keep up with her family and friendships—much less make it through a day teaching elementary school.

When a menstrual cycle lasted three months, she was diagnosed with uterine fibroids and ovarian cysts. She rejected the suggestion by her gynecologist to take cancer medication or have a hysterectomy and decided instead to try BHRT. However, the treatments given by the first doctor she consulted only worsened her problems. "They turned me into a bloated zombie," Maria said. "I was looking for signature treatment and felt I was getting cookie-cutter medicine."

Her sister-in-law, a happy patient of Dr. George Arnold, told her to give Signature Hormones a try. "Dr. Arnold listened to all my health concerns and addressed each one," said

Maria. "He examined all my previous lab tests and compared them to his own. He took the time to explain the test results, listened to my questions, and then explained what he was prescribing and why."

Dr. Arnold changed Maria's progesterone dosage and added thyroid. Then he added in a range of vitamins and mineral supplements and put her on a gluten-free diet. At her first checkup, Maria's bloodwork was improved and her fibroids had shrunk. Today, her menstrual cycle is normal.

"My former self has been reawakened," Maria said, adding that her energy and concentration have returned, and her confidence "is through the roof." Today, she is a school administrator who has an active family and social life. "With Dr. Arnold, I got what I was looking for—a treatment that is designed for what I need, based on science."

TREATING WITH ESTROGEN

For women who still have a uterus, estrogen supplements should always be accompanied by progesterone supplements. Traditionally, only Provera (a progestin and not real progesterone) was recommended for women with a uterus based on the idea that the uterus was the primary home of progesterone receptors. Women who no longer had a uterus were typically given estrogen alone. However, as you now know, progesterone receptors reside throughout your body and are involved in many body functions, not just the uterus.

Just as there can be an imbalance in estrogen and progesterone when your body is still producing these, there can be an imbalance in replacing estrogen and progesterone as well. That is why it is so important to ensure that the right balance is present. Among the problems of prolonged use of progesterone without adequate estrogen is increased appetite and cravings for carbohydrates, ultimately leading to increased fat storage and weight gain. Too much progesterone without estrogen can lead to bloating and gas because of Candida overgrowth. Candida is yeast that lives in your mouth and gut, helping with your digestion and nutrient absorption. Constipation or incontinence, and even the formation of gallstones, may also be caused by progesterone without estrogen.

Prolonged use of progesterone without adequate estrogen increases the bad cholesterol in your body (LDL) and decreases the good cholesterol (HDL).

When progesterone supplements are taken without estrogen, your triglyceride and cortisol levels can rise. Depression and fatigue can set in, and you can begin to lose your desire for sex. When progesterone is taken without estrogen, your muscles struggle to manage your body's glucose, which can lead to insulin resistance.[61]

When estrogen doesn't accompany progesterone in HRT, growth hormone levels can lower. Growth hormone stimulates growth and aids in cell reproduction and regeneration. Oral estrogen may also reduce IGF-1, a protein that helps build muscle.

While many believe that bioidentical progesterone in cream form offers no protection against cancer of the uterus, there is some evidence to show that it does. In a study in which twenty-six women completed treatment of either an oral dose of estrogen plus an oral dose of progesterone, or an oral dose of estrogen plus a progesterone

---

61   S. Kumagai, A. Holmäng, and P. Björntorp, "The effects of oestrogen and progesterone on insulin sensitivity in female rats," *Acta Physiologica* 149, no. 1 (September 1993): 91-7, accessed on National Library of Medicine National Institutes of Health, November 22, 2016, https://www.ncbi.nlm.nih.gov/pubmed/8237427.

cream, 77 percent preferred estrogen plus the cream.[62] And none of the participants were found to have signs of cancer in the uterus.

Estrogen taken by mouth raises sex-hormone-binding globulin (SHBG) levels, which results in lower testosterone levels. Oral estrogen may reduce lipid oxidation—the breakdown of fats in the blood—after meals and lead to a reduction in lean mass and an increase in fat mass.

Oral estrogen can raise liver enzymes, since 40 to 60 percent of the dose is extracted by the liver, and your liver does not need all that hormone. Elevated liver enzymes leak into the bloodstream and may indicate damage to the liver.

Estrogen given by mouth can interrupt the conversion of trypto-phan, an essential amino acid, into the mood-regulating neurotrans-mitter serotonin, which converts to melatonin. I'll talk about the benefits of melatonin in chapter 7.

Oral estrogen can also raise estrone, which as I mentioned earlier can potentially include the risk of breast and uterine cancer when levels are too high. Taking estrogen orally may also raise your blood pressure and triglycerides (body fat), and it can increase C-reactive protein, an indicator of inflammation in the body.

Taking estrogen by mouth increases your risk four fold of developing a blood clot. Oral estrogen is associated with an increased risk of venous thromboembolism, a blood clot in a deep vein, commonly the leg. Especially in patients at risk for Factor 5 Leiden, an inherited blood-clotting condition, estrogen is best administered transdermally (through the skin as a patch or cream). In these patients, studies have

---

62   H. B. Leonetti, et al., "Transdermal progesterone cream as an alternative progestin in hormone therapy," *Alternative Therapies in Health and Medicine* 11, no. 6 (November-December 2005): 36-8, abstract accessed on National Library of Medicine National Institutes of Health, November 10, 2016, https://www.ncbi.nlm.nih.gov/pubmed/16320858.

found that blood clots occur because of oral estrogen's effect on the liver, which doesn't occur when the hormone is applied transdermally.

It bears repeating: Clinical studies show that the increased risk of developing breast cancer occurs when using a combination of estrogen and progestin—not because of the estrogen, but because of the progestin Provera, which is the synthetic form of progesterone.

While transdermal estrogen in a patch or cream is the preferred form offered by Signature Hormones, there are exceptions to the rule. I have had patients who were unable to absorb estrogen through the skin, either by patch or cream, and their symptoms only responded to estrogen given orally. When transdermal doesn't work, the option to take estrogen orally does exist.

DISPELLING THE MYTHS OF ESTROGEN

Unfortunately, there is still a lot of misconception about HRT. When asked about HRT and which hormone can increase the risk of breast cancer, most women reply "estrogen."

Since estrogen has such an impact on the brain, many of the questions or comments that I get from patients center around brain function. Typical comments include:

Q: "I think I'm losing my mind."

A: You're not losing your mind, but you may have an estrogen imbalance. Estrogen increases blood flow to the brain. It also protects neurons and regulates the use of glucose and oxygen by brain cells. It has a significant effect on neurotransmitters, which affect your mood, memory, and mental state.[63]

---

63   G. Fink, et al., "Estrogen control of central neurotransmission: effect on mood, mental state, and memory," *Cellular and Molecular Neurobiology* 16, no. 3 (June 1996): 325-44, abstract accessed on National Library of Medicine National Institutes of Health, November 22, 2016, https://www.ncbi. nlm.nih.gov/pubmed/8818400.

Q: "I have lost the ability to spell."

A: Estrogen helps keep your brain healthy and sharp by keeping your blood-brain barrier operating effectively.

Q: "I can't remember where I parked my car."

A: Low estrogen levels can make you feel as if you have the onset of dementia or problems with concentration and focus. Estrogen also increases the availability of the neurotransmitter acetylcholine, which is related to memory and motor functions.

Q: "I am always dropping things."

A: Estrogen aids in manual speed and dexterity, and helps raise your body's sensitivity to nerve growth factor (NGF), a protein that helps develop and stabilize sensory neurons.

ESTROGEN IS A PROBLEM FOR MEN

In men, high levels of estrogen can be an especially difficult problem.

As men age, their levels of estrogen rise due to increased aromatase activity, which is the conversion of testosterone to estrogen. In the male body, estrogen is produced from testicular and adrenal androgen precursors. Precursors are the hormones earlier in the sequence when one hormone transforms into another; androgens are the male sex hormones. So, remarkably, estrogen is synthesized from testosterone!

Like women, estrogen in men is essential for brain function and cardiovascular and bone health. However, when estrogen levels are high in a man, the result can be less bioavailable testosterone. Other problems associated with high estrogen levels in men include:

- reduced libido

- reduced muscle tone

- increased fat tissue

- gynecomastia (male breasts)

- higher risk of diabetes, heart attack, benign prostatic hypertrophy, and some cancers

In men, estradiol—the strongest and most prominent form of estrogen—has a high affinity for bone estrogen receptors, which results in the stimulation of osteoblasts, leading to increased bone remodeling.

Elevated estrogen levels in men can also occur as a result of:

- obesity

- alcohol use

- altered liver function

- zinc deficiency

- estrogen imbalance caused by some drugs

- ingestion of xenoestrogens from the environment

So, it's crucial to monitor estrogen levels in men considering testosterone-replacement therapy.

LISA NEEDED A BIT MORE

Lisa was extremely pleased with her results—her hot flashes had cleared, her night sweats had stopped, and she was sleeping soundly again. However, her sex drive had not changed, so we added in testosterone administered in cream form. When the cream didn't deliver the results she desired, we switched the route of administration to injectable testosterone. She experienced a huge improvement in symptoms along with more normalized testosterone levels almost immediately.

Like some patients, Lisa also noticed relief for other symptoms that she had not initially reported to me. She had improved clarity of thought after she first began treatment. Often, following initial treatment, patients find that other issues they hadn't considered to be related problems were in fact being caused by hormone imbalances.

Chapter 6 Symptom Chart: **Testosterone**

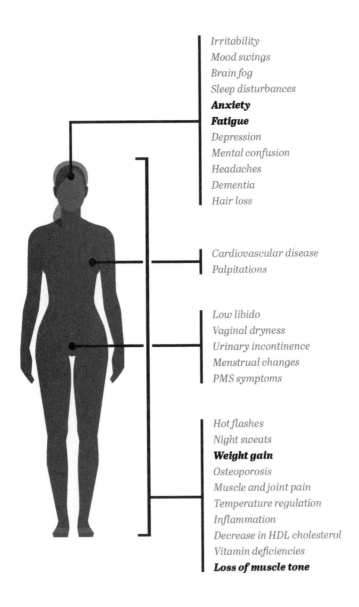

Irritability
Mood swings
Brain fog
Sleep disturbances
Anxiety
Fatigue
Depression
Mental confusion
Headaches
Dementia
Hair loss

Cardiovascular disease
Palpitations

Low libido
Vaginal dryness
Urinary incontinence
Menstrual changes
PMS symptoms

Hot flashes
Night sweats
Weight gain
Osteoporosis
Muscle and joint pain
Temperature regulation
Inflammation
Decrease in HDL cholesterol
Vitamin deficiencies
Loss of muscle tone

Chapter 6

TESTOSTERONE: NOT JUST "A MALE THING"

In her mid-fifties, Sam had already been "feeling her age." She'd been dealing with what she decided were probably symptoms of menopause—hot flashes, night sweats, and increasing moodiness. Then she began feeling more fatigued and was having a lot of trouble maintaining her concentration at work, changes she chalked up to what had become a sporadic sleep pattern, at best. When her hair started thinning at an alarming rate, she went to see her family physician, who offered no solution and just wanted to prescribe a sedative to help her sleep at night.

No matter how much she maintained her workout schedule, Sam was losing muscle tone and mass. To make matters worse, she was finding it difficult to concentrate on one task, let alone more—a matter that was beginning to affect her life both at home and at work. When her libido all but disappeared, she came to see me.

I started Sam on a low dose of testosterone cream, and within a few weeks, she felt "like a renewed woman."

WOMEN GET "LOW T," TOO

It's surprising to many women that low testosterone isn't a "male-only" condition. If you're a member of "The Best-Me Club," then you may know exactly what it feels like to have low levels of testosterone, a.k.a. Low T.

The symptoms of Low T in women can include:

- muscle wasting

- weight gain

- fatigue

- low self-esteem

- decreased HDL

- dry, thin skin with poor elasticity

- thinning and dry hair

- droopy eyelids

- sagging cheeks

- thin lips

- anxiety

Testosterone is produced in the ovaries and the adrenal glands, those two thumb-size organs above your kidneys that are involved in producing dozens of hormones to keep your body humming along. Most of the testosterone in your body comes from these two sources.[64]

Testosterone is produced by precursor hormones, one of which is androstenedione, which is a steroid hormone. Most androstenedione converts to estrogen (in the form of estrone), although some of it

---

64   T. C. Luoma, "The Female Low-Testosterone Epidemic," *T Nation*, August 5, 2014, accessed November 8, 2016, https://www.t-nation.com/training/female-low-testosterone-epidemic.

converts to testosterone. A powerful example of the effect of andro-stenedione can be seen in female hyenas during pregnancy, when an overabundance of androstenedione converts to testosterone to the point that female pups are born with genitals that resemble those of the males of the species. [65]

Women have less total testosterone than men—0.7–3.6 pg/dl compared to 0.95–4.3 pg/dl in men—and free or unbound testosterone values are 6–86 ng/dl compared to 270–1100 ng/dl in men. What constitutes "deficient" when it comes to normal levels of female testosterone? Free testosterone levels under 25 ng/dl in women up to age fifty years is generally considered low.

Men make, on average, eight to ten times more testosterone than women, but women are far more sensitive to the effects of testosterone. In other words, a little testosterone goes a long way. And yet, healthy women have testosterone levels that are ten times greater than the levels of estrogen in their bodies.[66]

As a matter of general practice, doctors don't commonly measure testosterone levels in women. If you go to your doctor with worries about excess scalp hair loss, midlife acne, or sprouting facial hair, your doctor may test for elevated levels of testosterone. But looking for any opportunity to supplement your levels of testosterone is not typically on the doctor's radar.

WOMEN AND TESTOSTERONE

Most people know testosterone as a sex hormone. As a "Best-Me Club" member, you may have already felt a surprising dip in your sex drive. In menopause, your ovaries stop producing testosterone. By

---

65   T. C. Luoma, "The Female Low-Testosterone Epidemic," *T Nation*, August 5, 2014, accessed November 8, 2016, https://www.t-nation.com/training/female-low-testosterone-epidemic.

66   Ibid.

the time you're postmenopausal, you may have half the testosterone you had when you entered it.

Still, half of women ages eighteen to fifty-nine report a lack of sex drive. Maybe you're one of those women who has noted a lower sex drive as part of a laundry list of symptoms, only to be discounted by your family physician who suggests you go "see someone for counseling." Instead of needing someone to examine what's going on in your head, what you're really dealing with is a hormone imbalance. And testosterone deficiency is a key part of that imbalance.

In fact, if you're still ovulating, you may have experienced an increase in your desire to have intercourse during ovulation. A rise in your testosterone level is responsible for that.[67] Testosterone combines with estrogen—which is produced in your body's fat tissues—to help grow, maintain, and repair reproductive tissues.

Testosterone and estrogen also affect other body tissues and bone mass. Osteoporosis—another component to membership in "The Best-Me Club"—may be prevented by healthy levels of testosterone.

Estrogen and testosterone work with calcium-regulating hormones to regulate the growth of your skeleton. In early puberty, estrogen helps increase bone growth. Near the end of puberty, a high concentration of estrogen and testosterone ends bone growth, determining a person's height.[68]

Testosterone is important for skeletal growth, both because of its direct effects on bone and its ability to stimulate muscle growth, which increases bone formation. As a stimulator of muscle growth, testosterone helps increase bone formation. In chapter 5, I talked

---

67   T. C. Luoma, "The Female Low-Testosterone Epidemic," *T Nation*, August 5, 2014, accessed November 8, 2016, https://www.t-nation.com/training/female-low-testosterone-epidemic.

68   Department of Health and Human Services, Office of the Surgeon General, *Bone Health and Osteoporosis: A Report of the Surgeon General* (Rockville, Maryland, 2004), accessed on National Library of Medicine National Institutes of Health, November 10, 2016, https://www.ncbi.nlm.nih.gov/books/NBK45513/pdf/Bookshelf_NBK45513.pdf.

about how bones are continually transforming through resorption, a natural remodeling process involving a balance of osteoclasts and osteoblasts. Declining testosterone levels affect the osteoclast/blast balance, negatively impacting the integrity of the skeleton and increasing the risk for fracture and compression fractures of the spine.[69]

Studies conducted on men found that testosterone improved muscle mass by increasing protein synthesis, and it's generally believed that the same occurs in women.[70] Protein synthesis is a biological, cell-building process that helps rebuild muscle tissue. During exercise, muscles incur tiny tears at the cellular level. Protein synthesis helps repair those tears by increasing blood flow to the area.[71] For protein synthesis to occur, you need sufficient amounts of testosterone, growth hormone, and protein in your body. Growth hormone, which is naturally produced in the pituitary gland, helps maintain human tissue by regenerating cells.[72] The good news is that lifting weights is one natural way to raise testosterone levels, although HRT can boost your efforts at the gym.

Now, I'm not talking about testosterone in the form of anabolic steroids, which many athletes and bodybuilders use. When misused, anabolic steroids can lower high-density lipoprotein cholesterol levels

69   Xu Feng and Jay McDonald, "Disorders of Bone Remodeling," *Annual Review of Pathology Mechanisms of Disease* 6 (2011): 121-145, accessed on National Library of Medicine National Institutes of Health, November 10, 2016, https://www.ncbi.nlm.nih.gov/pmc/articles/PMC3571087/.

70   R. C. Griggs, et al., "Effect of testosterone on muscle mass and muscle protein synthesis," *Journal of Applied Physiology* 66, no. 1 (January 1989): 498-503, abstract accessed on U.S. National Library of Medicine National Institutes of Health, November 10, 2016, https://www.ncbi.nlm.nih.gov/pubmed/2917954.

71   Stephanie Crumley Hill, "Protein Synthesis in Muscle Growth," *Livestrong.com,* December 21, 2015, accessed November 10, 2016, http://www.livestrong.com/article/179888-protein-synthesis-in-muscle-growth/.

72   Paul Roberts, "Human Growth Hormone: Everything You Need to Know about HGH," *Muscle & Fitness,* accessed November 10, 2016, http://www.muscleandfitness.com/supplements/build-muscle/everything-you-need-know-about-human-growth-hormone.

(HDL), which is, again, the "good" cholesterol that protects against heart disease.

Improving muscle tone is especially important for women who suffer from leaky bladder, a problem that occurs for many women in menopause. Leaky bladder (stress urinary incontinence) occurs when pelvic muscles lose their tone. For many women, regaining strength and tone in the pelvic muscles is achieved through a prescribed application of testosterone cream coupled with a regular program of Kegel exercises.

Testosterone also increases a sense of emotional well-being in women. According to a study in *Mauritas, the European Menopause Journal*, women suffer from depression more often than men, a factor that is directly related to testosterone levels in plasma.[73]

Testosterone elevates norepinephrine (noradrenaline), which, as I discussed in chapter 2, is part of the fight-or-flight mechanism of the brain. As a stress hormone, norepinephrine affects parts of the brain where attention and responding actions are controlled. Elevating norepinephrine helps your attention span by increasing your mind's ability to focus while blocking out distractions from external sources.[74]

In postmenopausal women, testosterone replacement helps maintain memory. In a recent study of women given a placebo or a testosterone gel, verbal learning and memory improved in those who received the treatment versus the placebo.[75]

---

73 U. D. Rohr, "The impact of testosterone imbalance on depression and women's health," *Maturitas* 41, Supplement 1 (April 2002): S25-46, supplement accessed on U.S. National Library of Medicine National Institutes of Health, November 8, 2016, https://www.ncbi.nlm.nih.gov/pubmed/11955793.

74 "Ritalin packs punch by elevating norepinephrine, suppressing nerve signal transmissions," American Physiological Society, news release, *EurekAlert.org* (May 30, 2006), accessed November 10, 2016, https://www.eurekalert.org/pub_releases/2006-05/aps-rpp052206.php.

75 "Testosterone Improves Verbal Learning and Memory in Postmenopausal Women," Endocrine Society, news release, accessed November 10, 2016, https://www.endocrine.org/news-room/press-release-archives/2013/testosterone-improves-verbal-learning-and-memory-in-postmenopausal-women.

For those of you who have managed to lose weight during menopause despite hormonal imbalances, testosterone can even help with sagging skin. Sagging occurs because the skin has expanded in areas where you've stored extra fat, and as it expands, skin tends to lose some or all of its elasticity. Not everyone who loses weight ends up with sagging skin. And other factors can compound the problem—genetics, your age, where the fat was stored, and how long you carried it around. [76]

Now, there is much debate about whether another androgen hormone in your body—dihydrotestosterone (DHT)—is beneficial or what some call the "evil twin" of testosterone. High levels of DHT are believed to be the culprit for hair loss, and in men, may be behind prostate cancer. DHT is a more potent and active androgen in your body than testosterone. It is made from testosterone, converted via the enzyme 5 alpha-reductase (5-AR). The body is loaded with androgen receptors that house concentrations of the 5-AR enzyme. Unlike testosterone, DHT does not aromatize (convert) into estrogen. [77]

Sex-hormone-binding globulin (SHBG), which moves the sex hormones DHT, testosterone, and estrogen through your bloodstream to be used by your body's cells, has a greater affinity for DHT and testosterone than it does for estrogen. Again, higher levels of SHBG lead to less available testosterone. [78]

Interestingly, men who become fathers experience a significant drop in their testosterone levels. According to a study of more than six hundred men in Cebu City, Philippines, rising cortisol levels in new

76   Chris Shugart, "Loose Skin: The Facts," *T-Nation.com*, February 16, 2016, accessed November 10, 2016, https://www.t-nation.com/diet-fat-loss/loose-skin-the-facts.

77   V. A. Randall, "Role of 5 alpha-reductase in health and disease," *Baillière's Clinical Endocrinology and Metabolism* 8, no. 2 (April 1994): 405-31, abstract accessed on U.S. National Library of Medicine National Institutes of Health, November 11, 2016, https://www.ncbi.nlm.nih.gov/pubmed/8092979.

78   Kalyn Weber, "Sex Hormone Binding Globulin: What Every Woman Should Know," *Inside-Tracker* (August 12, 2014), accessed November 11, 2016, https://www.insidetracker.com/blog/post/94531931309/sex-hormone-binding-globulin-what-every-woman-should#.

fathers can lead to a suppression of testosterone.[79] As I mentioned in chapter 2, cortisol is known as the "stress hormone." The study found that men who care for children during the day may see an increase in cortisol levels, leading to a decrease in testosterone production.

Another cause of low testosterone levels in women is chemo-therapy, a common treatment for breast cancer.[80] Chemo can also lower estrogen and progesterone levels, and the disruption in your hormones can lead to loss of interest in sex.

Adrenal fatigue, which I discussed in chapter 2, can lead to Low T. When the hormone cortisol rises as the result of chronic stress, it suppresses the pituitary gland's ability to function well, which ultimately leads to Low T.[81] Depression and psychological trauma can also lower testosterone levels in women, again, due to external stressors that raise hormones such as cortisol.[82] Medications taken for these conditions, such as Prozac or Zoloft, alter the serotonin, or "feel good" transmitters, in the brain, which can interfere with the bioavailability of testosterone.

If you're one of the millions of women who suffer from endo-metriosis, you're indisputably a member of a subchapter of "The Best-Me Club." It's estimated that some 6–10 percent of women of reproductive age suffer from endometriosis, an often-painful disorder where endometrial cells—cells normally found in the lining

---

79   Lee T. Gettler, Thomas W. McDade, and Christopher W. Kuzawa, "Cortisol and testosterone in Filipino young adult men: evidence for co-regulation of both hormones by fatherhood and relationship status," *American Journal of Human Biology* 23, no. 5 (September-October 2011): 609-20, accessed on U.S. National Library of Medicine National Institutes of Health, November 11, 2016, https://www.ncbi.nlm.nih.gov/pubmed/21638512, doi: 10.1002/ajhb.21187.

80   "Loss of Libido," *Breastcancer.org*, accessed November 11, 2016, http://www.breastcancer.org/tips/intimacy/loss_of_libido.

81   Bryan Walsh, "The Truth About Adrenal Fatigue," *T Nation.com* (March 2, 2010), accessed November 11, 2016, https://www.t-nation.com/supplements/truth-about-adrenal-fatigue.

82   Berit Brogaard, "Depression and High Testosterone in Women," *Livestrong.com* (December 17, 2015), accessed November 11, 2016, http://www.livestrong.com/article/494945-depression-and-high-testosterone-in-women/.

layer inside the uterus—grow *outside* of the uterus.[83, 84] A 2014 study found that serum testosterone was significantly lower in women who had endometriosis.[85]

Hyperinsulinemia, a condition in which there are excess levels of insulin in the blood, can cause a lowering of testosterone levels, but testosterone replacement can decrease hyperinsulinemia. In men, one study found that low levels of testosterone play some role in the development of type 2 diabetes.[86]

Birth control pills are one of the causes of Low T. Birth control pills cause a decline in testosterone, because they inhibit adrenal production of testosterone and they raise SHBG levels, which as I mentioned, decrease the amounts of free testosterone in your blood. In fact, the increase in SHBG has been found to lower free testosterone levels by twice as much as total testosterone levels.[87]

The lower the free testosterone in your body, the more likely you are to develop coronary artery disease. Testosterone improves exercise-induced ST depression—a sign of coronary artery obstruction—by dilating coronary arteries. Low testosterone is also associated with dyslipidemia, which is an elevation of LDL, or "bad" cholesterol.

83 "How many people are affected by or at risk for endometriosis?" *Eunice Kennedy Shriver National Institute of Child Health and Human Development*, accessed November 11, 2016, https://www.nichd.nih.gov/health/topics/endometri/conditioninfo/pages/at-risk.aspx.

84 Mayo Clinic Staff, "Endometriosis," *Mayo Clinic.org*, accessed November 11, 2016, http://www.mayoclinic.org/diseases-conditions/endometriosis/home/ovc-20236421.

85 Yoshihiro J. Ono, et al., "A Low-Testosterone State Associated with Endometrioma Leads to the Apoptosis of Granulosa Cells," *PLoS One* 9, no. 12 (December 23, 2014), accessed on U.S. National Library of Medicine National Institutes of Health, November 11, 2016, https://www.ncbi.nlm.nih.gov/pubmed/25536335.

86 R. K. Stellato, et al., "Testosterone, sex hormone-binding globulin, and the development of type 2 diabetes in middle-aged men: prospective results from the Massachusetts male aging study," *Diabetes Care* 23, no. 4 (April 2000): 490-4, abstract accessed on U.S. National Library of Medicine National Institutes of Health, November 11, 2016, https://www.ncbi.nlm.nih.gov/pubmed/10857940.

87 Y. Zimmerman, et al., "The effect of combined oral contraception on testosterone levels in healthy women: a systematic review and meta-analysis," *Human Reproduction Update* 20, no. 1 (2014): 76-105, accessed on U.S. National Library of Medicine National Institutes of Health, November 11, 2016, https://www.ncbi.nlm.nih.gov/pmc/articles/PMC3845679/.

As with other hormone tests, "normal" may not be the best indicator of Low T—you may be experiencing the symptoms of Low T regardless of what your lab tests reveal. The best measure of testosterone is free testosterone, or bioavailable testosterone. The free testosterone available in your body is only about 1 percent of the total. Eighty percent of the testosterone in a healthy woman's body binds to SHBG, while the remaining 19 percent binds to albumin (protein). The albumin-bound testosterone and free testosterone are biologically active, meaning they are available for your tissues to use.[88] By weighing your symptoms against lab results, we can get the best idea of how to move forward with treatment.

KAREN

A Return to Youth

In her fifties, Karen found herself tired all the time and struggling to deal with the stresses of a large, busy family and a job that she loved. "I felt weak, exhausted, and old," she said. As a musical conductor, voice teacher, and sound healer, Karen began to cut back on her hours at work because her symptoms affected her ability to sing. She was putting on weight, and her hair began to thin; she lost her desire for intimacy, and depression set in to the point that she pulled away from others and began to be a recluse.

Then a friend told Karen about Dr. George Arnold, who diagnosed her with adrenal fatigue. He prescribed a line of adrenal supplements along with estrogen cream and oral pro-

---

88 Mohamed Yahya Abdel-Rahman, , "Androgen Excess," *Medscape.com*, August 1, 2016, accessed November 11, 2016, http://emedicine.medscape.com/article/273153-overview.

gesterone. Once her estrogen and progesterone levels were back in balance, Karen began using testosterone cream.

As a result, Karen reported she regained her health; her energy, hair, and sex drive returned. "I look and feel much younger," she said. "Dr. Arnold literally saved me. He has patience and great insight and skill. I'm not sure what would have become of me had I not found him."

SYMPTOMS OF ELEVATED TESTOSTERONE

Just as Low T can cause problems, so can too much testosterone—and some of the symptoms are the same whether your testosterone imbalance is low or high.

Too much testosterone in a woman can lead to masculinization, or virilization, which is the development of male characteristics. The obvious male characteristic that some women with high levels of testosterone experience is unwanted hair growth.

However, there are other, less visible symptoms of high testosterone that may cause you to seek help.

Among the symptoms of high testosterone is anxiety, a result of hormonal imbalance caused by changes in your body and lifestyle. Menopause, pregnancy, or times of high stress can change the levels of estrogen and testosterone in your body, leading to feelings of anxiousness.

Too much testosterone can lead to feelings of agitation and anger, and the resulting frustration and inability to resolve such feelings can even lead to depression.

When too much testosterone causes oily facial skin, the result can be midlife acne—another source of frustration that can compound a woman's ire. Acne, however, can be an indicator of a bigger issue than just excess testosterone—a condition known as polycystic ovarian syndrome (PCOS).[89] In PCOS, the surface layer of the ovary is thick and it is hard for eggs to be released, so they accumulate under the surface, giving rise to multiple small cysts being seen on an ultrasound. Left untreated, PCOS can lead to infertility, diabetes, heart disease, or stroke.[90]

Sudden weight gain is another symptom of high testosterone levels. Alarming as an unexplained tightening of your pants can be, it's not always something you can easily control and, like acne, may indicate something more serious is going on inside, including PCOS, a tumor of the ovaries or adrenal gland, or the congenital disease adrenocortical hyperplasia. These conditions impact your adrenal glands, causing them to signal the production of more hormones from the ovaries that develop into testosterone.[91] A dysfunction of the adrenal gland leading to high testosterone levels may also cause you to crave salt and sugar.

One of the most serious risks of high testosterone levels is insulin resistance, which interferes with your body's ability to regulate its blood-sugar levels. Insulin resistance can lead to adult-onset diabetes, increasing your risk for heart disease, breast cancer, and uterine cancer.

89   Rachael Rettner, "Acne in Women Can Signal Hormone Problems," *Live Science.com* (November 27, 2012), accessed November 11, 2016, http://www.livescience.com/25049-women-acne-hormone-disorder.html.

90   Maureen Salamon, "Polycystic Ovary Syndrome: Symptoms and Treatment," *Live Science.com* (May 28, 2013), accessed November 11, 2016, http://www.livescience.com/34805-pcos-symptoms-treatment-insulin-resistance.html.

91   Rachel Nall, "High Testosterone in Women & Weight Gain," *Live Strong.com* (August 16, 2013), accessed November 11, 2016, http://www.livestrong.com/article/315045-high-testosterone-in-women-weight-gain/.

A supraphysiologic dose of testosterone, or a dose that is larger or more potent than a naturally occurring dose, increases insulin resistance.

TREATMENT FOR LOW/HIGH TESTOSTERONE

Traditional testosterone-replacement therapy can involve oral administration, a transdermal cream, transdermal gel, or intramuscular injection. At Signature, your customized testosterone treatment starts with a bioidentical testosterone cream. In some people, the cream will not produce the desired results, and a bioidentical testosterone injection will be required.

When it comes to correcting Low T levels, we may also administer doses of bioidentical estrogen when needed, since estradiol must be optimized for testosterone replacement to perform at its best. Without enough estrogen, testosterone cannot attach to brain testosterone receptors.

For patients with elevated testosterone, we offer three forms of bioidentical therapies:

- **Saw palmetto**, which is made from the berries of a palm-like plant that is prevalent in the southeastern United States.

- **Glucophage (metformin)**, a slow-release form of a blood-glucose-lowering medication that improves insulin sensitivity with few side effects.

- **Spironolactone**, which significantly lowers plasma testosterone levels.

In addition to testosterone-replacement therapy, there are other ways to raise testosterone levels, including:

- Decrease your calorie intake.

- Increase the amount of protein in your diet.

- Take the amino acids arginine, leucine, and glutamine.

- Exercise.

- Get enough sleep.

- Lose weight.

- Reduce your external stressors.

In addition to a healthy diet, zinc is shown to increase testosterone levels, especially in males that are deficient in the mineral. Vitamin B6 and magnesium also aid in zinc absorption and the converting of free cholesterol to testosterone.

DISPELLING THE MYTHS OF TESTOSTERONE

Here are some of the misconceptions I hear from patients about testosterone-replacement therapy.

Q: "Will I grow big, bulky muscles?"

A: No. However, at the low amounts of testosterone you will be getting, your muscles will have better tone and definition.

Q: "Will I become overly aggressive?"

A: Levels of testosterone that are *too high* can cause aggressive personality changes. Again, we start low and monitor to ensure your dosage is accurate for you.

Q: "Doesn't testosterone-replacement therapy cause cancer?"

A: Testosterone administered at low doses does not increase the risk for breast cancer in women. In men, there has been ongoing debate about whether testosterone replacement will increase prostate cancer risk. The FDA warns that prostate cancer is a clear contraindication for testosterone replacement.[92] However, a recent study found that the incidence of prostate cancer is not increased by testosterone replacement.[93] Testosterone does not cause prostate cancer, and there is no evidence that testosterone replacement accelerates BPH (benign prostatic hypertrophy).[94]

AND NOW, THE MALE PART

Of course, testosterone is a male hormone, and yet just like women, a man's testosterone levels decline because of the aging process. In fact, a man's testosterone levels peak in his mid-twenties and then start a gradual decline, at which point symptoms begin to arise. By age forty, a man's testosterone levels decline naturally by 1 percent each year. By ages fifty to seventy, half of healthy men will have bioavailable levels of testosterone below the lowest levels found in healthy men who are twenty to forty years old.[95]

In a man, testosterone is a sex hormone, and there are testosterone receptors all over a man's body. Testosterone is involved in the making of protein and muscle formation. It also helps manufacture bone and improves oxygen uptake throughout the body.

92 "Testosterone supplementation after prostate cancer?" Harvard Medical School + Harvard Health Publications, *Prostate Knowledge*, accessed November 11, 2016, http://www.harvardprostateknowledge.org/testosterone-supplementation-after-prostate-cancer.

93 "Testosterone therapy does not raise risk of aggressive prostate cancer," *Science Daily. com* (May 7, 2016), accessed November 11, 2016, https://www.sciencedaily.com/releases/2016/05/160507143326.htm.

94 J. E. Morley, "Testosterone replacement and the physiologic aspects of aging in men," *Mayo Clinic Proceedings*, supplement. doi 75(2000):S83-7.

95 S. G. Korenman, et al., "Secondary hypogonadism in older men: its relationship to impotence," *The Journal of Clinical Endocrinology & Metabolism* 71 (1990): 963-969, accessed on U.S. National Library of Medicine National Institutes of Health, November 11, 2016, https://www.ncbi.nlm.nih.gov/pubmed/2205629.

Proper levels of testosterone in a man's body help control blood sugar, regulate cholesterol, maintain a powerful immune system, aid in mental concentration, improve mood, and protect the brain against Alzheimer's disease.

In chapter 1, I talked about andropause, the male version of menopause. To expand on that discussion, here is a more extensive list of the symptoms of andropause:

- fatigue, tiredness, or loss of energy
- depression, low or negative mood
- irritability, anger, or bad temper
- anxiety or nervousness
- loss of memory or concentration
- loss of sex drive or libido
- loss of erections or problems during sex
- decreased intensity of orgasms
- backache, joint pains, or stiffness
- loss of fitness
- feeling overstressed
- decrease in job performance
- decline in physical abilities
- bone loss
- elevated cholesterol

Testosterone-replacement therapy for men is safe and can provide significant benefits. Transdermal testosterone is 81 percent effective in resolving issues with erectile dysfunction. Oral testosterone treatments are 51 percent effective. And intramuscular injections (IMs) are 53 percent effective.[96]

Other benefits of testosterone-replacement therapy include improved mood and interest in sex.[97]

Testosterone replacement also prevents the production of beta-amyloid precursor protein in men, which may protect against Alzheimer's disease.[98]

The lower the total testosterone, free testosterone, and bio-available testosterone in a man's body, the more likely the presence of coronary artery disease.[99] Testosterone improves exercise-induced ST depression—a sign of a coronary artery obstruction—by dilating coronary arteries. Low testosterone is also associated with an elevation of LDL, or "bad" cholesterol.[100]

And, as I mentioned earlier, studies have found that the incidence of prostate cancer is not increased by testoster-

---

96   P. Jain, A. W. Rademaker, and K. T. McVary, "Testosterone supplementation for erectile dysfunction: results of a meta-analysis," *The Journal of Urology* 164, no. 2 (August 2000): 371-5, abstract accessed on U.S. National Library of Medicine National Institutes of Health, November 11, 2016, https://www.ncbi.nlm.nih.gov/pubmed/10893588.

97   G. M. Alexander, et al., "Androgen-behavior correlations in hypogonadal men and eugonadal men. Mood and response to auditory sexual stimuli," *Hormones and Behavior* 33, no. 2 (1998): 85-94, abstract accessed on U.S. National Library of Medicine National Institutes of Health, November 11, 2016, https://www.ncbi.nlm.nih.gov/pubmed/9154431.

98   G. K. Gouras, G, et al., "Testosterone reduces neuronal secretion of Alzheimer's beta-amyloid peptides," *Proceedings of the National Academy of Sciences U.S.A.* 97, no. 3 (2000): 1202-5, on U.S. National Library of Medicine National Institutes of Health, November 11, 2016, https://www.ncbi.nlm.nih.gov/pubmed/10655508.

99   G. Rosano, et al., "Acute anti-ischemic effect of testosterone in men with coronary artery disease," *Circulation*, vol. 99, no. 13(April 6, 1999): 1666-70, abstract accessed on U.S. National Library of Medicine National Institutes of Health, November 11, 2016.

100 K. M. English, et al., "Men with coronary artery disease have lower levels of androgens than men with normal coronary angiograms," *European Heart Journal* 21, no. 11 (2000): 890-4, European Heart Journal, vol. 21, no. 11(2000):890-4

one replacement.[101] Testosterone-replacement therapy does not cause prostate cancer, and there is no evidence that testosterone replacement accelerates BPH (benign prostatic hypertrophy).[102]

Treatment for men includes transdermal bioidentical testosterone cream. The transdermal cream we use at Signature is specially made in a compounding pharmacy and is less expensive than using AndroGel testosterone gel. Your testosterone cream is formulated specifically for *you*.

TREATING THE MEN

In addition to treating the female Sam I mentioned at the start of this chapter, I've also got a couple of cases to share with you about males who received testosterone therapy through Signature. As a member of "The Best-Me Club," you may have a significant other who is going through changes brought on by aging who is also looking for relief (or perhaps you need the relief).

Do either of these stories sound like someone you know?

CASE #1: FIFTY-THREE-YEAR-OLD MEL

Mel was a fifty-three-year-old man who gradually developed symptoms over approximately five years that included decreased endurance, weight gain around the waist, irritability, decreased erections, loss of morning erection, morning sluggishness, low sex drive, increased

101   NYU Langone Medical Center, "Testosterone therapy does not raise risk of aggressive prostate cancer," *Science Daily.com* (May 7, 2016), accessed November 11, 2016, https://www.sciencedaily.com/releases/2016/05/160507143326.htm.

102   J. E. Morley, et al., "Testosterone replacement and the physiologic aspects of aging in men," *Mayo Clinic Proceedings*, supplement. doi 75(2000):S83-7.

seasonal allergies, fatigue, breast enlargement, grumpiness, muscle aches and stiffness, lack of enthusiasm, and a ringing in the ears. He had tried herbal remedies and found that they made his irritability worse and had no effect on any of his other symptoms. By the time he came to Signature, he had quit taking all his medications, having given up on finding a cure for his symptoms.

Hormonal testing revealed a normal hemoglobin level, normal thyroid function, low free testosterone, normal estradiol, and low DHEA. I started him on testosterone with Chrysin (a medication that prevents testosterone from being converted to estrogen) in a cream to be applied once a day, along with DHEA as a slow-release capsule taken by mouth once a day.

Two months after he started on his personalized regimen, he came in for a follow-up and was happy to report mental clarity, greater ability to handle stress, and a surge in energy. He had also lost nine pounds and was having morning erections along with an improved sex drive. His muscle aches and stiffness were almost gone, and his breast enlargement had reduced.

His lab testing showed an elevation in his testosterone levels, but also an increase in his DHEA and estrogen level. An elevation in a male's estrogen level when taking testosterone is an unwanted side effect that needs to be addressed. We kept the testosterone and DHEA dosages the same but increased the amount of Chrysin. This change successfully reduced his estrogen level back to a normal level.

CASE #2: THIRTY-SEVEN-YEAR-OLD DAVE

Just as women experience perimenopause as hormone levels start to decrease, men can also experience periandropause as hormone levels start to decrease.

Dave was thirty-seven years old when he came to me reporting that he had been under a lot of stress for the past two years. He had recently moved to Canada from the United States, gotten married, and then had a new child. His symptoms included increased anxiety and general irritability. He found himself overreacting to the smallest issues, just unable to handle problems. He also complained of decreased endurance, weight gain around the waist, decreased erections, a burned-out feeling, foggy thinking, memory lapses, morning sluggishness, low sex drive, fatigue, loss of his sense of humor, depression, muscle aches and stiffness, lack of enthusiasm, feeling pressed for time, poor exercise tolerance, and increased caffeine consumption.

He wasn't taking any medications when he came to see me. When I conducted lab testing on him, we found he had low testosterone and low DHEA but normal estrogen and hemoglobin levels. I diagnosed him with adrenal fatigue and low testosterone and DHEA. An individualized regimen consisting of treatment for adrenal fatigue, DHEA, and testosterone was created for Dave.

Two months later, he noted that he was handling stress much better and that his irritability was significantly improved. Lab testing showed his DHEA still low, so I increased his dosage. I also increased his testosterone dosage, because there was still room for improvement in some of his symptoms.

Another two months later he was "doing great." He had lost weight and had returned to a regular exercise routine at the gym where he was already building up muscle mass. When his labs came back with estrogen levels a little high, I increased his Chrysin level and asked him to return six months later.

Sam, Mel, and Dave are just three examples of patients who have found great success with testosterone-replacement therapy.

Now let's look at a hormone that is a building block for nearly all the hormones I've discussed so far—dehydroepiandrosterone, more commonly known as DHEA.

Chapter 7 Symptom Chart: **DHEA**

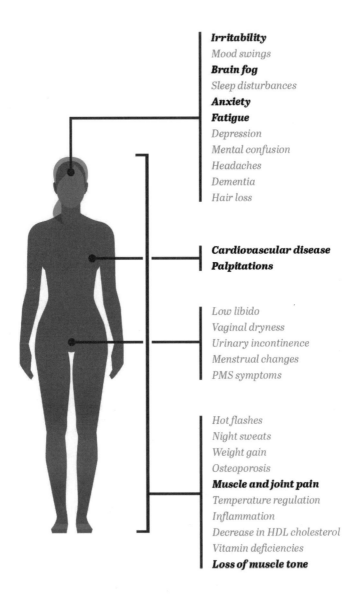

Irritability
Mood swings
Brain fog
Sleep disturbances
Anxiety
Fatigue
Depression
Mental confusion
Headaches
Dementia
Hair loss

Cardiovascular disease
Palpitations

Low libido
Vaginal dryness
Urinary incontinence
Menstrual changes
PMS symptoms

Hot flashes
Night sweats
Weight gain
Osteoporosis
Muscle and joint pain
Temperature regulation
Inflammation
Decrease in HDL cholesterol
Vitamin deficiencies
Loss of muscle tone

Chapter 7

DHEA: AN ESSENTIAL BUILDING BLOCK

Dehydroepiandrosterone (DHEA), also known as androstenolone, acts as a building block for the production of the sex hormones (androgens and estrogens) in both men and women. DHEA converts into estrogen and testosterone in both men and women. In men, it mainly converts into estrogen; in women, it mainly converts into testosterone.

A small amount of DHEA is made in the cells of your brain and skin, but most of it is made by the adrenal glands. Like other hormones in your body, production of DHEA declines with age. Starting in your late twenties, DHEA levels begin to diminish. By the age of seventy, your body may only make one-fourth of the amount of DHEA it made when you were younger.

Cholesterol is a precursor to the production of DHEA. DHEA is biosynthesized from cholesterol through a four-step process that begins with cholesterol entering the mitochondria of the cells. Mitochondria are rod-shaped, organized structures within cells that convert oxygen and nutrients into adenosine triphosphate (ATP), which are the cells' energy transporters. After cholesterol enters a cell, it is then converted to pregnenolone, a steroid hormone. Pregnenolone is then converted to 17-OH pregnenolone. Finally, 17-OH pregnenolone is converted to DHEA.[103]

DHEA is a versatile hormone, one that adapts readily to different situations and builds from other hormones. It helps protect against a wide range of conditions.

The heart and vascular system are prime beneficiaries of good levels of DHEA. It lowers serum cholesterol, particularly LDL, or "bad," cholesterol, which can cause blockages when it collects on the walls of your blood vessels.[104] DHEA may improve overall blood-vessel function, decreasing the formation of fatty deposits in your blood vessels and preventing blood clots from forming.

One study found that DHEA significantly improved epithelial cell function.[105] Epithelial cells line blood-vessel walls and aid in the ability of the vessels to contract and dilate. The study also found that DHEA supplementation restored epithelial cell health, helping to lower the release of plasminogen activator inhibitor type 1 (PAI-1) protein. PAI-1 keeps tiny blood clots that continually form in your bloodstream from dissolving. Undissolved clots can eventually form larger clots that can block blood flow, leading to a condition known as thrombosis. When epithelial cells are unhealthy, they allow PAI-1 to be released unchecked.

103 W. L. Miller, "Early steps in androgen biosynthesis: from cholesterol to DHEA," *Baillière's Clinical Endocrinology and Metabolism* 12, no. 1 (April 1998): 67-81, abstract accessed on U.S. National Library of Medicine National Institutes of Health, November 11, 2016, https://www.ncbi.nlm.nih.gov/pubmed/9890062.

104 J. Christopher-Hennings, et al., "The effect of high fat diet and dehydroepiandrosterone (DHEA) administration in the rhesus monkey," *In Vivo* 9, no. 5 (September-October 1995): 415-20, abstract accessed on U.S. National Library of Medicine National Institutes of Health, November 11, 2016, https://www.ncbi.nlm.nih.gov/pubmed/8900917.

105 Aaron W. Jensen, "DHEA Protects Against Heart Disease and Diabetes," *Life Enhancement.com*, accessed November 12, 2016, http://www.life-enhancement.com/magazine/article/875-dhea-protects-against-heart-disease-and-diabetes.

DHEA can affect how insulin works in your body. Studies have shown DHEA to be effective in reducing insulin resistance.[106]

Bone thinning can occur when DHEA is depleted, which as I mentioned can happen when cortisol levels are high. DHEA can help supply the hormones needed to facilitate bone resorption, stimulating new bone-cell formation while breaking down old bone. In a study of 225 healthy adults ages fifty-five to eighty-five, a 50 mg daily oral supplementation of DHEA for one year saw modest improvement in bone-mineral density (BMD).[107]

In weight loss, the benefits of DHEA may come largely from its conversion to testosterone, which can help rid the body of fat while negating estrogen's fat-storing tendencies.[108] DHEA supplements can also alter your body composition by promoting weight loss and increasing lean muscle mass.

Like testosterone, DHEA can improve brain function. With DHEA, better brain function comes from the hormone's protective effects against high cortisol levels.

As an inflammation-lowering hormone, DHEA is a friend to your overall immune system. Inflammation is one cause of heart disease, involving your body's cytokines—those protein molecules that stimulate cells to respond to sites of inflammation, trauma, and infection in your body. DHEA can lower some of the cytokines that

---

106   Edward P. Weiss, et al., "Dehydroepiandrosterone (DHEA) replacement decreases insulin resistance and lowers inflammatory cytokines in aging humans," *Aging* 3, no. 5 (May 2011): 533–542, accessed on U.S. National Library of Medicine National Institutes of Health, November 24, 2016, https://www.ncbi.nlm.nih.gov/pmc/articles/PMC3156603/.

107   D. Von Mühlen, et al., "Effect of dehydroepiandrosterone supplementation on bone mineral density, bone markers, and body composition in older adults," *Osteoporosis International* 19, no. 5 (May 2008): 699-707, accessed on U.S. National Library of Medicine National Institutes of Health, November 12, 2016, https://www.ncbi.nlm.nih.gov/pmc/articles/PMC2435090/, doi: 10.1007/s00198-007-0520-z.

108   J. Buvat, "Androgen therapy with dehydroepiandrosterone.," *World Journal of Urology* 21, no. 5 (November 2003): 346-55, abstract accessed on U.S. National Library of Medicine National Institutes of Health, November 12, 2016, https://www.ncbi.nlm.nih.gov/pubmed/14551720.

stimulate inflammation.[109] DHEA has been shown to inhibit inter-leukin-6 (IL-6), a pro-inflammatory cytokine, while promoting the release of interleukin-2 (IL-2), a cytokine that regulates white blood cells.[110]

The issues of decline that come with aging have been associated with an increase in IL-6 and a decline in DHEA and IL-2. People suffering from the effects of rheumatoid arthritis, lupus, HIV and AIDS, trauma, and sepsis have been found to have lower levels of DHEA.[111] Taking a DHEA supplement has been clinically proven to help restore hormone blood levels in people feeling the effects of stress, aging, and a compromised immune system.[112] A study using supplements of 7-keto DHEA found that this DHEA metabolite improved the immune system, lowered diastolic blood pressure, and increased white blood cells in elderly women and men.[113] These activities help the body maintain and repair itself and can even reduce allergic reactions. A study looked at DHEA supplementation as a possible solution for asthma and found that it was effective in suppressing type 2 helper T cells (Th2), which join with other cells to trigger allergic inflammation.[114]

---

109   "DHEA: Surviving and Thriving," Women's International Pharmacy *Connections*, accessed November 12, 2016, http://www.womensinternational.com/connections/dhea.html.

110   F. Hammer, et al., "Sex steroid metabolism in human peripheral blood mononuclear cells changes with aging," *The Journal of Clinical Endocrinology & Metabolism* 90, no. 11 (November 2005): 6283-9, accessed on U.S. National Library of Medicine National Institutes of Health, November 13, 2016, https://www.ncbi.nlm.nih.gov/pubmed/16091484.

111   C. C. Chen and C. R. Parker Jr., "Adrenal androgens and the immune system," *Seminars in Reproductive Medicine* 22, no. 4 (November 2004): 369-77, abstract accessed on U.S. National Library of Medicine National Institutes of Health, November 13, 2016, https://www.ncbi.nlm.nih.gov/pubmed/15635504.

112   G. Valenti, "Neuroendocrine hypothesis of aging: the role of corticoadrenal steroids," *Journal of Endocrinological Investigation* 26, supplement 6 (2004): 62-63, abstract accessed on U.S. National Library of Medicine National Institutes of Health, November 13, 2016, https://www.ncbi.nlm.nih.gov/pubmed/15481804.

113   J. Zenk and M. Kuskowski, "The use of 3-acetyl-7-oxo-dehydroepiandrosterone for augmenting immune response in the elderly," paper presented at meeting of Federation of American Societies for Experimental Biology (FASEB), April 17, 2004.

114   Yong Cui, et al., "Effects of Combined BCG and DHEA Treatment in Preventing the Development of Asthma," *Immunological Investigations* 37, no. 3 (2008): 191-202, abstract accessed on U.S. National

DHEA can also lower triglycerides, which can lead to heart disease, diabetes, and fatty liver.

HIGH/LOW DHEA

As with any hormone, too much DHEA isn't going to do you any favors. DHEA is a powerful hormone, and too much of it can cause symptoms ranging from fatigue and restless sleep to mood changes and irritability to depression and anger. The goal with DHEA, as with all hormones, is *balance*—DHEA needs to work with the other hormones in your body. Results with DHEA supplementation can vary from person to person since it's such a complex hormone, so it's important to start with a lower dose and then come in for follow-up to monitor your levels.

Many of the symptoms of excess DHEA stem from the fact that it's converted to other sex hormones in your body. For that reason, DHEA supplements are not for women who are pregnant or expect to get pregnant soon. Since DHEA can increase estrogen, which can in turn increase the growth of breast-cancer cells, DHEA is not for women being treated for breast cancer. And since lowering testosterone is one treatment for prostate cancer, men with that disease should not take DHEA.

Since DHEA is an essential building block, when it is low, it can impede the body's ability to produce other hormones. When your DHEA levels are low, you may experience a range of symptoms including irritability and higher levels of stress, less energy and muscle strength, lower tolerance for infections, joint soreness, and weight gain.

Library of Medicine National Institutes of Health, November 13, 2016, https://www.ncbi.nlm.nih.gov/pubmed/18389439, doi: 10.1080/08820130801967833.

There are several causes of low DHEA: for starters, menopause—your admission ticket into "The Best-Me Club"—is a primary reason that your DHEA levels will begin to decline. Also, as your body ages, production of DHEA naturally declines. Smoking—one factor you *can* control—may cause a drop in DHEA, because nicotine inhibits the production of 11-beta-hydroxylase, an enzyme produced by the adrenal glands that is needed to make DHEA.

The upside of replacing DHEA means you can enjoy:

- increased muscle strength and lean body mass

- an activated immune system

- less stress

- better sleep

- an overall feeling of wellness

- less joint pain

- better sensitivity to insulin

- lower triglycerides

When you visit our office, testing of your hormones will be completed by blood, urine, or saliva. That's right, we can measure your DHEA levels from a sample of your saliva. We then treat with an oral capsule or sublingual drops, which have been shown to be more effective than transdermal creams.

Women are more sensitive to the effects of DHEA supplementation and therefore need less DHEA than men. For a woman, a dose up to 15 mg of DHEA is typically enough. However, if the DHEA is being prescribed for rheumatoid arthritis, then higher doses may be needed. Since men metabolize DHEA at a faster rate than women, a dosage of 25 to 50 mg is more appropriate.

A final note on DHEA: When cortisol and DHEA levels decline, they can lead to the condition I've discussed earlier—adrenal fatigue, also known as adrenal burnout.

ADRENAL BURNOUT

I've talked about how adrenal glands control your body's stress-response center. When your adrenal glands aren't functioning properly, you're more susceptible to illness and allergies. When your body needs to deal with a stressful situation, the hormones released by the adrenals send the signals that get your body to act on the perceived threat. When you're under constant real or perceived threat—such as a stressful job, a family situation, or maybe a chronic disease—your adrenals have trouble keeping up with all the energy you need. The result is adrenal fatigue, or adrenal burnout.

As I discussed in chapter 2, adrenal fatigue is an important matter to address when looking at HRT.

If you're experiencing full-on adrenal burnout, then you're likely having some of these symptoms:

- fatigue
- low blood pressure
- sensitivity to light
- insomnia
- digestive problems
- emotional imbalances/lack of motivation
- hypoglycemia
- hypothyroidism that does not respond to treatment
- decreased immunity
- lack of stamina
- emotional paralysis
- poor wound healing
- allergies
- alcoholism and drug addiction
- decreased sexual interest
- feeling of being overwhelmed

Adrenal fatigue is a middle-ground, of sorts, between two more serious diseases—Cushing's Syndrome and Addison's Disease. While adrenal fatigue can lead to life-altering complications such as high blood pressure, diabetes, and depression, Cushing's and Addison's can be life-threatening without the proper treatment. Addison's develops when the adrenal glands don't produce enough cortisol. That happens when the signal the brain sends to the adrenals to produce cortisol is disrupted. Cushing's is the result of too much cortisol, which is typically caused by a tumor of the pituitary or adrenal glands.

Treating adrenal fatigue involves using a mix of vitamins, adaptogenic herbs, and replacing DHEA. The DHEA in high-quality supplement capsules comes from the compound diosgenin, which comes from wild yams.

Adaptogenic herbs are herbal medicines used for centuries to restore health and vitality and improve stamina and immunity. Adaptogens help regulate your adrenal response system by increasing energy while instilling calm. Adaptogens also have antioxidant and anti-inflammatory effects that can protect your cells. Adaptogens get their name from their ability to adapt to your specific needs. In addition to adaptogens, I may prescribe organic adrenal extracts, a natural hormone replacement backed by more than ninety years of research. I may also have you take licorice (Glycyrrhiza Glabra), a root with antidepressant compounds that decrease the amount of hydrocortisone broken down by the liver. That action reduces the demand on the adrenals to produce more cortisol.

SHEILA

Hope When It Seemed There Wasn't Any

Following a laparoscopic hysterectomy, Sheila initially seemed to be recovering well. But after a few months, she began to have a number of symptoms—weakness, faintness, heart palpitations, muscle pains in her chest and back, restlessness, headaches, loss of appetite, digestive problems, anxiety and panic attacks, and fatigue. She battled the symptoms for more than two years, but with tests from her general practitioner showing "normal" results, no treatment was given. Her condition deteriorated to the point that she was barely able to function. "I'd make the bed and then have to lie down in it," she said. "I was so weak and fatigued, I felt like I was dying."

Then her general practitioner mentioned bioidentical hormone-replacement therapy (BHRT) as a possible solution. After researching BHRT online, she found George Arnold, MD, and Signature Hormones.

On her first visit, Dr. Arnold prescribed a cream to help with Sheila's low estrogen, progesterone, and testosterone levels. Without any real improvements, she was then prescribed DHEA and adrenal-support supplements to deal with her adrenal fatigue. Still, her symptoms did not improve. She had little appetite, she was too weak to care for her home and family, and her persistent heart palpitations had her in the emergency room more than once. She continued the treatment on Dr. Arnold's assurances, and in time, she began to improve. "I was finally able to walk into Dr. Arnold's office on my own, without leaning on my husband for support," Sheila said, adding that, with treatment, her adrenal glands were revived and are now working on their own.

"Dr. Arnold gave me hope when I thought there wasn't any," Sheila said. "I found him exceptionally caring, compassionate, patient, and reassuring. He always took time to address my concerns, and I always felt like he cared about my well-being. I'm truly blessed to have him as my doctor."

CORTISOL—THE STRESS HORMONE

Cortisol is the only hormone in the body that increases with age. As you grow older, your cortisol levels naturally rise. As I discussed in chapter 2, cortisol is a steroid hormone made by the adrenal glands, and it is secreted based on signals from the hypothalamus in the brain. When under stress, the body makes cortisol at the expense of DHEA, and over time, cortisol gradually depletes DHEA.

Normal cortisol levels are high in the morning and then taper off by the end of the day. That normal cycle of secretion is what's known as a "cortisol curve."

When you're stressed, your cortisol levels elevate, which is why it has been dubbed "the stress hormone." However, while that elevation is supposed to be a temporary situation, in today's 24/7/365 world, cortisol doesn't always lower right away.

When you're chronically stressed, the cortisol in your body doesn't taper off. Instead of being like a time-release pill giving you energy and focus on waking, waning over the course of the day, and then wearing off by bedtime, an overstressed body continues to release cortisol day and night. That leaves your body with too much cortisol, and all that excess cortisol leads to adrenal burnout. Too much cortisol can give you a wired-but-exhausted feeling. That can keep you awake at night, deplete the chemicals your brain and body need to function well, and cause your body to store fat, particularly in the midsection.[115]

Besides factors that induce stress, depression can also lead to abnormal cortisol cycling such as cortisol levels that are elevated all day or all night. High intake of progestin, or synthetic progesterone, can also lead to elevated cortisol levels.

Since most of your body's cells have cortisol receptors, when your levels are too high or too low, you'll feel the effects of adrenal fatigue. For instance, if you find yourself catching every cold you encounter, you may be dealing with an imbalance of cortisol levels, because too much cortisol can impede your immune system. If you're feeling so tired you drop into bed but so wired when you get there that you can't sleep, your cortisol levels may be out of whack. If your waistline is expanding despite more stringent calorie counting, you may have a cortisol problem. If you're having a heated discussion at 10:00 p.m. right after a light night workout, you may be on a cortisol roller coaster. All these symptoms and more can be caused when your cortisol levels don't function as they should—starting high in the morning and then dropping slowly throughout the day.

There are several conditions associated with abnormal cortisol levels.

For instance, during menopause, the adrenal glands produce estrogen and progesterone to take up some of the slack of diminishing production of these hormones from the declining ovaries. Unfortunately, the adrenal glands' task becomes more arduous when they

---

115 Elizabeth Millard, "The Cortisol Curve," *Experience Life*.com (March 2016), accessed November 14, 2016, https://experiencelife.com/article/the-cortisol-curve/.

are also working to pump out cortisol. In the struggle to determine which should take priority—stress hormones or sex hormones—cortisol tends to win out. As a member of "The Best-Me Club," the fact is that you need estrogen and progesterone to feel well as your body undergoes changes.

High levels of cortisol may be especially damaging to cardiovascular health. One six-year study of more than eight hundred people ages sixty-five and older found that cortisol increased cardiovascular mortality risk. For some, the risk was five times higher.[116]

Over the long term, elevated cortisol can also lead to higher blood sugar levels, since cortisol produces glucose as part of the fight-or-flight response to a stressor. Since cortisol's role is to render your cells resistant to insulin, chronically elevated cortisol levels can place great demand on the pancreas as it struggles to provide an endless stream of insulin to normalize your body's glucose. Meanwhile, your blood glucose levels remain high, potentially damaging your organs, and yet your cells are still starved for the sugar energy they need.

High levels of cortisol have also been found to have potentially damaging effects on the adult brain. A six-year study of more than four hundred adults—those whose brains had high levels of cortisol, along with high levels of the protein amyloid beta, which is associated with Alzheimer's disease—saw greater memory decline than study participants with low levels of cortisol.[117]

In addition to menopause, cardiovascular health, insulin resistance, diabetes, memory loss, and Alzheimer's disease, abnormal

---

116 Nicole Vogelzangs, et al., "Urinary Cortisol and Six-Year Risk of All-Cause and Cardiovascular Mortality," *The Journal of Clinical Endocrinology & Metabolism* 95, no. 11 (November 2010): 4959-4964, accessed on U.S. National Library of Medicine National Institutes of Health, November 14, 2016, https://www.ncbi.nlm.nih.gov/pmc/articles/PMC2968721/.

117 Merrillees, Louise, "Alzheimer's disease study finds potential link between stress hormone and speed f decline," *ABC News* (Australia, October 13, 2016), accessed November 14, 2016, http://www.abc.net.au/news/2016-10-13/research-shows-possible-link-between-cortisol-and-alzheimers/7930728.

cortisol levels have been associated with several other conditions, including:

- depression
- sleep disorders
- panic disorders
- infertility, impotence
- anorexia nervosa
- PMS
- osteoporosis
- rheumatoid arthritis
- IBS (inflammatory bowel disease)
- exacerbations of multiple sclerosis
- breast cancer
- chronic fatigue syndrome (CFS)
- fibromyalgia

Since cortisol normally peaks early in the morning and then tapers off by evening, the best way of measuring your cortisol levels is with a four-sample saliva test that we conduct throughout the day.

One way to rein in cortisol and control adrenal fatigue is by replacing necessary nutrients with a one-a-day vitamin containing:

- vitamin C
- B vitamins
- calcium
- magnesium

- zinc

- selenium

- copper

- sodium

- manganese

Other supplements that can get your cortisol levels under control include phosphatidylserine, a type of molecule found in your body's cells. Phosphatidylserine is highly concentrated in your brain cells, where it aids in the activity of neurotransmitters such as acetylcholine, which is related to memory and motor function, and dopamine, which regulates movement and emotional responses. Phosphatidylserine also lowers cortisol levels, fuels the brain by boosting brain-glucose metabolism, and enhances the activity of nervous-system molecules. Research has shown that phosphatidylserine supplementations can deter—and potentially even reverse—dementia- or age-related cognitive declines in memory, mood, learning, and concentration.[118]

Fish-oil supplements—omega-3 fatty acids containing eicosapentaenoic acid (EPA) and docosahexaenoic acid (DHA)—also bring relief for cortisol imbalances and adrenal fatigue. EPA and DHA when consumed together can help support memory and concentration, keep triglyceride levels healthy, promote better metabolism of fat and cholesterol, and give you an overall sense of well-being.

Cortef, or hydrocortisone, is an adrenocortical steroid that can relieve allergic or breathing disorders, skin conditions, ulcerative colitis, arthritis, lupus, and psoriasis.

---

118   P. M. Kidd, "A review of nutrients and botanicals in the integrative management of cognitive dysfunction," *Alternative Medicine Review* 4, no. 3 (1999): 144-61, abstract accessed on U.S. National Library of Medicine National Institutes of Health, November 13, 2016, https://www.ncbi.nlm.nih.gov/pubmed/10383479.

Stress-reduction techniques can help you maintain a sense of calm in the face of whatever stressor comes your way. Your adrenal glands pump out cortisol regardless of the type of stress you're encountering—physical or mental. Finding ways to regain control in the face of any type of perceived threat is the way to keep your cortisol levels in check. Daily walks, meditation, yoga, prayer, or other relaxation techniques can help keep your nervous system centered throughout the day, and when employed in the evening, can help you sleep better at night.

PREGNENOLONE—A PRECURSOR HORMONE

Like DHEA, pregnenolone is a steroidal hormone your body manufactures. Pregnenolone is a precursor hormone to DHEA; it converts into DHEA.

Pregnenolone is synthesized from cholesterol. This synthesis occurs primarily in the adrenal glands, though it is made in other areas of your body as well, including your liver, brain, and ovaries as well as your skin and even in your eye retinas. If your cholesterol levels are too low, you may not be able to make pregnenolone effectively—and that can be a real problem.

You see, pregnenolone has numerous properties that protect your cells and promote better health. Unfortunately, like DHEA, pregnenolone levels decline with age. At age seventy-five, most people have 65 percent less pregnenolone than they had at age thirty-five.

Pregnenolone's function in the body is to regulate the balance between excitation and inhibition in the nervous system. It increases resistance to stress and improves energy both physically and mentally.

Pregnenolone modulates the neurotransmitter gamma-aminobutyric acid (GABA), which sends chemical messages throughout your brain and nervous system. GABA calms activity in your nerve cells, helping you relax and control your fear and anxiety when neurons become overexcited. Pregnenolone also modulates N-methyl-D-aspartate (NMDA) receptors. NMDA is involved in learning, memory, and alertness. When you're mentally sluggish or feeling depressed, chances are you're dealing with excessive GABA activity and decreased NMDA activity. Benzodiazepine drugs such as Valium or Xanax, which are often prescribed for anxiety, depression, panic attacks, or other such conditions, activate GABA receptors. Pregnenolone, on the other hand, inhibits GABA receptors, lowering their activity while raising NMDA activity—elevating mood and making pregnenolone a natural antidepressant and stress reducer.

As a GABA blocker, pregnenolone also helps keep your brain sharp. It helps to repair nerve damage by promoting the formation of the protective layer known as the myelin sheath that surrounds many nerve-cell fibers. Pregnenolone can also improve sleep, and its ability to reduce inflammation and block acid-forming compounds makes it an excellent pain regulator.[119]

Like the other hormones in your body, too much pregnenolone can have negative effects. One of the most visible of these is acne, which is believed to occur because pregnenolone converts to androgens. Too much pregnenolone supplementation can cause drowsiness, but it can also cause insomnia if you become overstimulated. Low levels of pregnenolone can help you relax, but high levels can make you more prone to becoming irritable, angry, or anxious. One side effect of too much pregnenolone supplementation is headaches.

Even doses of pregnenolone as low as 5 mg per day can cause heart palpitations, which can be a serious issue in some people.

119   "Pregnenolone: Scientific View and Its Outweigh Benefit," NDRI.com, accessed March 27, 2017, http://ndri.com/article/pregnenolone_scientific_view_and_its_outweigh_benefit-412.html.

People may also suffer from fluid retention and muscle aches with pregnenolone supplementation.

In addition to the aging process, there are several reasons a person may be dealing with low pregnenolone. These include eating too many saturated fats and trans fats, which can block the pathways to pregnenolone production. Having cholesterol levels that are too low (yes, there is a point where cholesterol can be too low) can lead to low pregnenolone, since pregnenolone is made from cholesterol. Hypothyroidism, or low thyroid, can lead to low pregnenolone levels, as can a tumor of the pituitary gland. And if you have a severe illness or other trauma, pregnenolone will pump out the cortisol to help the body deal with stress while making less of the other hormones your body needs.

Overall fatigue, muscle weakness, and arthritic joint aches and pains can indicate pregnenolone deficiency, since the hormone fights inflammation. Since pregnenolone is a mood elevator, depression may be a symptom of a deficiency. Low pregnenolone can leave you with insomnia, a lack of focus, and the inability to deal with stress. And since pregnenolone is ten times more concentrated in the brain than in the blood, deficiencies can lead to impaired memory.

At Signature, we look at pregnenolone for treating moodiness and depression; memory loss; sleep disturbances; and autoimmune diseases such as rheumatoid arthritis, lupus, and ankylosing spondylitis—a disease that causes fusing of spinal vertebrae.

MELATONIN—MORE THAN JUST A SLEEP AID

Melatonin—which you may have heard of as a natural sleep aid—is another helpful hormone produced in your body and one that decreases in levels as you age.

Melatonin is made in your pineal gland (an endocrine gland in your brain), retina, gastrointestinal tract (GI), and in your white blood cells (WBCs). Melatonin decreases cortisol levels, helping to calm you in the face of stressors you encounter throughout the day.

Beyond being a sleep aid, melatonin is a powerful antioxidant, because it quells inflammation, which aids the immune system.

Melatonin also helps prevent cancer by blocking estrogen's tendency to bind to breast cells and stimulate cancer growth.

Melatonin as a supplement encourages sleep by lowering the body temperature and blood pressure and inducing prolonged REM sleep.[120] As a sleep-aid supplement, melatonin helps prevent insomnia in people trying to discontinue the use of benzodiazepines, which are often prescribed for anxiety.[121] Abrupt discontinuation of benzodiazepines often results in side effects including anxiety and insomnia, which can be barriers to discontinuation among long-term users. Melatonin improves the onset, duration, and quality of sleep.

Melatonin deficiencies are derived from various sources, among which is alcohol consumption. Although beer and wine contain melatonin, studies have found that consuming alcohol can actually lower melatonin levels.[122] As a stimulant, caffeine's effects are the opposite of melatonin, which can decrease melatonin levels. Tobacco

120   D. J. Dijk and C. Cajochen, "Melatonin and the circadian regulation of sleep initiation, consolidation, structure, and the sleep EEG," *Journal of Biological Rhythms* 12, no. 6 (December 1997): 627-35, abstract accessed on U.S. National Library of Medicine National Institutes of Health, November 16, 2016, https://www.ncbi.nlm.nih.gov/pubmed/9406038.

121   A. Wright, et al., "The Effect of Melatonin on Benzodiazepine Discontinuation and Sleep Quality in Adults Attempting to Discontinue Benzodiazepines: A Systematic Review and Meta-Analysis," *Drugs & Aging* 32, no. 12 (December 2015): 1009-18, abstract accessed on U.S. National Library of Medicine National Institutes of Health, November 15, 2016, https://www.ncbi.nlm.nih.gov/pubmed/26547856.

122   Katri Peuhkuri, Nora Sihvola, and Riitta Korpela, "Dietary factors and fluctuating levels of melatonin," *Food & Nutrition Research* 56 (2012), accessed on U.S. National Library of Medicine National Institutes of Health, November 15, 2016, https://www.ncbi.nlm.nih.gov/pmc/articles/PMC3402070/, doi: 10.3402/fnr.v56i0.17252.

may cause excess melatonin levels.[123] And exposure to weak electromagnetic fields may disrupt melatonin, as one study found, leading to long-term health effects.[124]

Medications may also interact with melatonin. The list of medications that may interact with melatonin includes, but is not limited to: antibiotics, aspirin, acetaminophen, birth control pills, diabetes medications, lansoprazole (Prevacid) and omeprazole (Prilosec) stomach medications, heart and blood pressure drugs, and blood-clot preventers.[125]

The actual dosage of melatonin can vary but should start with as little as 0.5 mg, and then work up to the ideal dose, typically not to exceed more than 5 mg. However, caution should be taken by patients with autoimmune disease, since melatonin can trigger the immune system, making autoimmune diseases worse. Other patients who should be cautioned before taking melatonin include those who are dealing with depression. Patients who should not take melatonin include pregnant or breastfeeding women, people taking steroids, and anyone dealing with lymphoma or leukemia.

As with many hormones, a little melatonin goes a long way. Excess melatonin can lead to symptoms such as headaches and depression. Daytime sleepiness and fatigue can result if melatonin is taken during the day or too high a dose is used.[126]

123 C. Ursing, et al., "Influence of cigarette smoking on melatonin levels in man," *The European Journal of Clinical Pharmacology* 61, no. 3 (May 2005): 197-201, accessed on U.S. National Library of Medicine National Institutes of Health, November 16, 2016, https://www.ncbi.nlm.nih.gov/pubmed/15824912.

124 M. N. Halgamuge, "Pineal melatonin level disruption in humans due to electromagnetic fields and ICNIRP limits," *Radiation Protection Dosimetry* 154, no. 4 (May 2013): 405-16, https://www.ncbi.nlm.nih.gov/pubmed/23051584, doi: 10.1093/rpd/ncs255.

125 Lynn Marks, "What Are Melatonin Supplements?" *Everyday Health.com*, accessed November 15, 2016, http://www.everydayhealth.com/drugs/melatonin.

126 A. Herxheimer, A. and K. J. Petrie, "Melatonin for the prevention and treatment of jet lag," *The Cochrane Database of Systematic Reviews* 2 (2002): CD001520, accessed on U.S. National Library of Medicine National Institutes of Health, November 16, 2016, https://www.ncbi.nlm.nih.gov/pubmed/12076414.

Some users have reported that melatonin causes vivid dreams and nightmares, which may be occurring upon waking quickly from the REM cycle when dreams are the most intense.[127]

Excess melatonin can also cause weight issues. It can disrupt cortisol levels, which can lead to more fat storage when cortisol mobilizes stored triglycerides, moving them to the fat cells in the abdomen—this is how you develop that spare tire. Excess melatonin also suppresses serotonin, a neurotransmitter that keeps carbohydrate cravings at bay.

Studies have also found that light exercise can raise melatonin levels, which can even offer protection against cancer.[128]

Several medications have been known to cause excess melatonin levels in your body, either by causing additional melatonin to be secreted or by causing your body to absorb more supplemental melatonin.

A number of foods can also cause excess melatonin production, including:

- bananas

- barley

- cherries

- ginger

- oats

- rice

- sweet corn

---

127 "Melatonin in Food and Wine," Sleepdex.org, accessed November 15, 2016, http://www.sleepdex.org/melatonin.htm.

128 University of Toronto, "Study Demonstrates Role Of Exercise In Modifying Melatonin Levels; Increase Believed To Offer Breast Cancer Protection," *Science Daily.com* (December 3, 2005), accessed November 15, 2016, https://www.sciencedaily.com/releases/2005/12/051202132144.htm.

- tomatoes

- walnuts

DISPELLING THE MYTHS OF DHEA

Here are some of the misconceptions I hear from patients about DHEA replacement therapy.

Q: "I've heard that DHEA is dangerous. Is that true?"

A: DHEA is a naturally occurring hormone. DHEA supplements are steroid hormones that are structurally related to testosterone and are designed to stimulate protein synthesis, muscle growth, and insulin. As with any hormone, giving too much can cause side effects. If too much DHEA is given, the most common side effects are acne and hair loss.[129]

Q: "Isn't DHEA for men only?"

A: As a precursor to all human sex hormones, DHEA can benefit women as well, helping to correct hormonal imbalances.

Q: "DHEA can't really combat all the effects of aging I'm feeling, can it?"

A: While it won't make you feel like you're twenty again, DHEA supplements can help correct your hormonal imbalances and combat many of the signs of aging you're feeling.

---

129   L. Anderson (medical reviewer), "Anabolic Steroids - Abuse, Side Effects and Safety," Drugs.com (May 04, 2014), accessed November 15, 2016, https://www.drugs.com/article/anabolic-steroids.html.

DHEA FOR MEN

DHEA can also help correct hormonal imbalance in men. DHEA levels in men begin to decline steadily after age thirty.

In men, DHEA can help protect against cardiovascular disease and can lower cholesterol levels. DHEA can also raise testosterone levels. Healthy levels of DHEA may help prevent atherosclerosis, or hardening of the arteries.

Chapter 8

HORMONE-REPLACEMENT THERAPY: A VISIT TO SIGNATURE

At the writing of this book, Courtney had been a client at my practice, Signature Hormones, for eight months. When she first came to see me, she was forty-seven years old and suffering from the symptoms of perimenopause: night sweats, insomnia, severe PMS, recurring yeast infections, increased susceptibility to illness, fatigue, and just an overall "run down" feeling.

Lab testing revealed she had low progesterone levels and was suffering from adrenal fatigue.

I put her on progesterone replacement and began treating her adrenal fatigue, and within two months her night sweats had ceased and her sleep had improved. On her first follow-up visit, she also reported a drop in her anxiety levels, which she hadn't even mentioned to me on her first visit. She felt better overall.

In a recent visit to me, Courtney remarked on how much she enjoyed visiting Signature. "Dr. Arnold," she said. "The most mean-ingful thing to me about your amazing office is that it's a safe place to speak up. I am not judged here." Courtney said that she had shared her symptoms with other women only to find them unsympathetic to her concerns. "I often find them judgmental," she said, "as if somehow I'm responsible for these symptoms I'm having. Since they aren't experiencing the same thing, then the problem must be me. ... I suffered in silence until coming to you."

Unfortunately, Courtney's experience is common. Some women sail through perimenopause and menopause with no symptoms at all, while others get more than their fair share of symptoms. Some women, I believe, continue to produce a small but significant amount of hormone that keeps their symptoms from showing in the first place. If we could figure out an easy solution to help all women sail through perimenopause and menopause, we'd bottle it up and make it available to everyone.

That, in a sense, is our goal at Signature Hormones. We want to help every woman who visits our practice relieve the bothersome symptoms in as natural a way as possible!

CONSULTATION AND FOLLOW-UP

Your visit to Signature Hormones starts with a friendly conversation, either via phone or e-mail, with one of my assistants. The goal is to put you at ease right from the start. The assistant outlines the process going forward, letting you know about hormone testing and what information needs to be collected to assist me in reaching a diagnosis for you. Then the assistant books your first consultation.

Prior to that first consultation, I typically have your complete lab testing so that when I see you, I can match what is happening hormonally with your symptoms.

However, as I've said throughout the book, it's never good to base your diagnosis and treatment solely on the numbers on a report. The numbers must be taken in context with what you are experiencing and living. That "big picture" is important and too-often missed by many physicians.

For instance, as I mentioned in chapter 2, with a problem like thyroid dysfunction, you may have classic signs and symptoms of an underactive thyroid gland, yet your lab test results are all "within the normal range." But you'll never overcome your problems if you don't get treated, because your lab tests are on the low or high end of the "normal" range. I've helped countless women by treating them after looking at the big picture instead of limiting my attention to numbers on a piece of paper.

At your consultation visit, you'll register with one of my assistants. You and I will then meet so I can learn more about your story. I'll spend most of our time together listening to you. I really need to hear about your symptoms, your life, your medical history. From the moment I ask, "How can I help you?" I want to give you as much time as it takes to tell your story in a safe, nonjudgmental environment.

As of this writing, I've seen nearly thirty thousand women and men in a career spanning more than thirty years. While at first you may be embarrassed to share the intimate details of your life, let me assure you that it's doubtful you'll bring in a story that will truly shock me. Please feel free to share; the more you tell me, the better I can help you. Again, I'm not here to judge. I'm here to help. Everything you share is kept in the strictest confidence.

After we talk, I sometimes conduct a physical examination. If it's needed, I explain what needs to be examined and why.

At the end of your visit, I put together all the information I've gathered, and then I discuss with your lab results with you. I look not only at lab results outside normal ranges but also what is within normal ranges to help me determine what you need based on what you have described to me.

As I mentioned in chapter 1, I will customize a prescription—to be specially compounded—based specifically on your unique needs. That prescription is very precise and includes the hormones I want you to take, the dosage and frequency, and the medium in which they are to be administered—either cream, capsule, troche (a soft, dissolvable disk), or liquid.

I can let you know on that first visit what treatment I think is best for you to correct any hormonal deficiencies along with what kind of results you should expect from your treatment.

Sometimes, multiple medications are required, but I limit how many we start at once. It can be a little overwhelming if too many treatments begin at the same time. And taking too many supplements at once can make it difficult to know what is working and what may need to be adjusted.

Your first follow-up should take place approximately eight weeks after starting your treatment. About two weeks prior to that visit, we'll have you do repeat lab testing.

At that first follow-up, you and I will review which symptoms are improved, and which, if any, have not. I compare your initial lab results with your most recent ones.

With all this information, I can get an objective measure of whether the medication is getting into your body and your body's response to it. I may adjust your medication, or add others, if needed.

Depending on how your body has responded to the medication, your next follow-up visit will be in either three months or six months. As always, if your symptoms change prior to your next visit, I encourage you to contact me. Typically, if there are any concerns, my assistant sends out a lab requisition to you, either by mail or e-mail, the results of which give me an objective assessment of your hormone levels.

My patients come from across Canada and outside the country. Some of my patients have difficulty organizing a trip to Markham, Ontario, to see me personally. In most of these cases, I can provide the same quality of service over the phone. Don't let the distance between us interfere with your decision to seek my help.

Whatever your location, filling your prescription is as close as a local compounding pharmacy. I work closely with reliable compounding pharmacies that ship not only locally but internationally as well.

As I mentioned in chapter 1, I have seen issues arise regarding the quality and consistency of hormone medication over time. I've built relationships with many pharmacists, which helps me recommend the best pharmacy for you: one that is close to you and will fill your prescription properly and that has the quality that I would want in a prescription for myself. Several of the pharmacies that provide service to my patients ship medication around the world.

FORM OF ADMINISTRATION

Hormones can work differently depending on the form of administration. Here are some of the hormones I've discussed in this book and the preferred form of administration:

- **Estrogen**. Estrogen given orally can have an adverse effect on your good and bad cholesterol levels and on the inflammatory pathway in your body. Estrogen given through the skin has a beneficial effect on your lipid profile and decreases inflammation in your body.

- **Thyroid**. Thyroid comes in oral form. It should be taken on an empty stomach, with no food consumed for one hour after the dose.

- **Testosterone**. Testosterone given by mouth can have a negative effect on your liver. Testosterone given by cream and by injection does not.

- **DHEA**. Current studies suggest that DHEA works better when given orally than via a cream.

- **Progesterone**. Progesterone given orally influences GABA receptors in your brain, which play a role in both quality and quantity of sleep—a major complaint of many women I see. Progesterone given via cream does not have the same effect as oral.

In my practice, I often see patients who have been treated by family physicians who have taken a weekend course in hormone treatment or by a pharmacist with no clinical experience.

When choosing a provider to help balance your hormones, look for one with the right training and experience, someone with a comprehensive knowledge of how different routes of administration can affect you.

DIFFERENT PATIENTS, DIFFERENT TREATMENTS

Here are some examples of patients I've seen that I think demonstrate what it means to visit Signature Hormones and receive treatment.

Jasmeen: No relief from her current practitioner.

Jasmeen is a sixty-eight-year-old woman referred to me by one of my colleagues. Jasmeen complained of hot flashes, heated episodes, heart palpitations, and mood changes. She also had high blood pressure and sporadic pelvic cramping.

Jasmeen had experienced an episode of vaginal bleeding, and a recent ultrasound and endometrial biopsy performed by her treating physician to look for a cause turned up nothing. She was taking a baby aspirin daily, two blood pressure medications, vitamins, and the traditional hormone-replacement medications Estrace, an estrogen, and Prometrium, a progesterone.

At Signature, her labs revealed her progesterone levels were ten times the norm!

I started Jasmeen on a customized program of bioidentical hormone replacement consisting of the estrogen cream Bi-Est—the cream composed of the weak estrogen estriol and the strong estrogen estradiol—in a ratio similar to what her ovaries used to produce. Jasmeen was also started on a sustained-release natural progesterone in a dose that was significantly lower than the Prometrium she had been receiving.

In a follow-up visit eight weeks later, Jasmeen reported that her cramping had settled and she had no further erratic bleeding episodes. Her energy and mood had improved. She was incredulous at the turnaround.

Repeat lab testing showed her progesterone level had returned to normal and her estradiol levels were up, even though the Bi-Est was delivering less estrogen than the Estrace she had been taking before.

I adjusted her prescriptions and asked her to return in six months, or to call if her symptoms changed in that time.

Jasmeen's story is not uncommon. Often, I see patients previously seen by other practitioners who have been unable to correct the underlying hormone imbalance.

David: Men need help, too.

What does a gynecologist know about male hormones? Well, in my case, a lot.

Men have the same hormones as women. Hormones in men occur in different amounts, but they have similar functions. I learned about men's needs after treating my female patients and then having them look to me for help in getting their male partners the same relief they experienced.

Fifty-five-year-old David is a good example. I had treated his wife for several years with excellent results. David had the classic symptoms of andropause: penis shrinkage, irritability, fewer erections, increased aggression, and poor exercise tolerance. His family physician had initially started him on AndroGel, a testosterone in gel form. David did not like the smell of the gel nor how much of it he had to lather on his body. He was switched to testosterone injections, which led to an unwelcome personality change.

At Signature Hormones, lab testing showed an elevated HbA1c (a plasma glucose measure over a three-month period), elevated triglycerides, elevated cholesterol, low DHEA, and one of the lowest total free-testosterone levels I have seen in a male.

I started David on DHEA, testosterone, and Chrysin, which is a bioflavonoid known to boost testosterone and inhibit its conversion to estrogen. I also prescribed other supplements to help with his abnormal lipid profile and elevated HbA1c. When David returned for his follow-up visit, not only had his andropause symptoms improved significantly, but his abnormal lipid profile and his elevated HbA1C were also improving.

David's case was a challenge because he had a lot of overlapping symptoms. Diagnosing a patient when similar symptoms arise from different sources is a challenge but one that I've encountered and overcome time and again. In doing so, I've often found other medical issues during a consult that a patient didn't realize he or she had. For instance, I've seen women and men with significant anemia that, once corrected, resolved *all* their symptoms. Diagnosing diabetes or prediabetes can lead to tremendous improvements in overall well-being and in weight-loss efforts. Hypothyroidism, once treated, leads to improved energy, improved mood, and weight loss.

At Signature, total body health is our goal. That's why we take a big-picture view of every patient rather than focus in on one symptom.

Crystal: Better quality of life.

At age forty-seven, Crystal came to me to improve her quality of life. She had no sex drive, intense PMS, inability to sleep, a stressful relationship with her husband, and was dealing with challenges concerning her twelve-year-old daughter. At the time, she was taking two antidepressants, but they were not providing any relief.

Lab testing showed elevated cholesterol and triglycerides, low vitamin B12, borderline HbA1c elevation, low thyroid function, and low levels of progesterone and testosterone.

I started Crystal on a natural, sustained-release progesterone capsule daily, testosterone cream, natural thyroid replacement, vitamin B12, and several supplements: vinpocetine, an anti-aging and cognitive function compound; ashwagandha, to soothe mental and physical stress; and 5-HTP, a serotonin enhancer.

Crystal returned to see me ahead of her scheduled follow-up visit because she was concerned that she was not improving. Repeat lab testing showed her hormone levels had improved, but since she was not experiencing corresponding improvement in her symptoms, I adjusted her medications.

Further questioning also revealed that Crystal had put on a lot of weight over the past several years, which made me look at her borderline HbA1c as a potential indicator of prediabetes or insulin resistance. She revealed to me that her family physician had also questioned whether she had diabetes, so I sent her for more tests, which revealed her fasting insulin was markedly elevated. I started her on a slow-release form of metformin, brand name Glumetza. Over the next several months, her insulin levels decreased, her energy improved, and she started losing weight.

Crystal's story demonstrates the importance of that big-picture view and also knowing when symptoms call for basic medicine.

Bruce: Taking a different route.

At age fifty-six, Bruce came to see me complaining of a lack of energy, generalized muscle aches and pains, and low sex drive. Lab testing revealed consistently low testosterone levels.

Bruce had tried testosterone cream before but had suffered through a flare of his inflammatory bowel disease as a side effect. Bruce was started on a low dose of testosterone in cream form and slowly increased the dose, keeping a careful eye on his colitis. Over the next few months, his testosterone cream was increased even more, and he did start to feel better but was still not getting the results he wanted.

I switched Bruce from cream to injections. Even though cream works better in most men, that's not the case for everyone.

After switching to injections, Bruce began feeling better, and his testosterone levels rose. I also had Bruce start taking the oral medication Arimidex to prevent the conversion of testosterone to estrogen. After starting Arimidex, Bruce's estrogen level dropped too low, which led him to feel unwell. I adjusted his medication, and his estrogen level returned to a more normal level, and he felt better.

As a result, Bruce began feeling fine. His colitis remained under control, and the symptoms he originally came to see me about all improved.

Like many of my patients, Bruce took accountability for his health by asking about how to better his health. When patients ask what medications to take, sometimes I don't know the answers and need to spend a little time researching the information they bring to me. But it's a challenge I enjoy—learning about new entries into the healthcare market and how they may help the people who come to see me.

HRT IS ABOUT BALANCE

Sometimes, after you start on HRT, your hormones may seem to be balanced, but then something happens and your symptoms return. Often, that simply means some adjustment of your medication. Sometimes other factors can trigger your hot flashes or other symptoms. For instance, hot flashes can be triggered by red wine, spicy foods, and stress.

If your symptoms return, consider whether one of these triggers or others are causing them. For instance, if you enjoy a glass of red wine, and it's followed by a hot flash, then you have a decision to make: If you can handle the symptom, then occasionally you may be okay with indulging in the trigger.

When it comes to stress, however, none of us is immune. Whenever possible, remove the stress trigger, because while balanced hormones can certainly help you deal with stress, no amount of medication can relieve all the symptoms of dealing with a chronically stressful situation.

Conclusion

Hormones in your body are interconnected—each hormone relies in some way on the function of another.

For instance, when your cortisol levels rise, your progesterone levels decrease, because cortisol competes with progesterone for common receptors. When your cortisol levels are elevated, more thyroid hormone is bound and is therefore less active.

All the hormones in the body are designed to work in concert with one another. No hormone works on its own. If one is altered, or deficient, it will affect the actions of all the other hormones. One size does not fit all when it comes to HRT. At Signature Hormones, we begin by identifying the underlying cause of your symptoms and then relieve your symptoms with natural, bioidentical hormones that feed your body's hormone receptors.

If you've been suffering in silence, it's time to speak up. You're not alone; you're part of a bigger community of women who want relief for their perimenopausal and menopausal symptoms.

Reach out to me and my team at Signature Hormones (www. georgearnoldmd.com) to schedule an appointment to talk about your symptoms and what can be done with hormone-replacement therapy to help you get your life back on track.

Bioidentical, compounded, customized hormone replacement is the only way to achieve and maintain the balance your body needs to feel your best and live your best—for life.

Our Services

Compassionate, individualized care delivered in an environment where you are safe to speak and not be judged.

Private confidential consultation for hormone imbalance, including perimenopause, menopause, depression during and after pregnancy, polycystic ovarian syndrome, thyroid dysfunction including both hypothyroidism (underactive thyroid function) and hyperthyroidism (overactive thyroid function), adrenal fatigue, low sex drive, and vaginal atrophy.

Consultations/follow-up visits provided in-office as well as by phone and online.

Men suffering from andropause.

Women who have had breast cancer suffering from menopausal symptoms.

Hormone testing.

Bioidentical hormone treatment programs customized specifically for you.

Follow-up hormone testing and follow-up assessments.

Non-hormonal laser treatment for vaginal dryness/burning/painful sex (especially helpful in women who have had breast cancer).